Overview of Target Cont
Total Intravenous
Second E........

Overview of Target Controlled Infusions and Total Intravenous Anaesthesia

Second Edition

Dr. Anthony R. Absalom
Consultant in Anaesthesia and Intensive Care
Addenbrookes Hospital
Cambridge, United Kingdom

Prof. Dr. Michel M. R. F. Struys
Professor in Anaesthesia and Research Coordinator
Department of Anaesthesia
University Gent
Gent, Belgium

ACADEMIA
PRESS

Uitgeverij Academia Press
Ampla House
Coupure Rechts 88
9000 Ghent
Belgium

www.academiapress.be

Academia Press is a subsidiary of Lannoo Publishers.

Anthony R. Absalom, Prof. Dr. Michel M. R. F. Struys
Overview of Target Controlled Infusions and Total Intravenous Anaesthesia
Gent, Academia Press, 2007, 108 p.

ISBN 978 90 382 1107 7
D/2007/4804/78

Notice
The author and publisher have carefully considered all drug dosages and therapies referred to in this book. However, neither the authors nor the publisher will be responsible for any patient harm caused by the clinical application or use of this book or the methods, processes or technologies identified, referred to or discussed in this book. You should seek professional/medical advice before attempting to seek to replicate any clinical application or use discussed in this book.

All rights reserved. No part of this publication may be reproduced, stored in a retrieval system, or transmitted in any form or by any means, electronic, mechanical, photocopying, recording or otherwise without the permission of the publishers.

Table of contents

GENERAL AND HISTORICAL BACKGROUND		5
I.	**TARGET-CONTROLLED INFUSIONS**	9
	1. Definition	9
	2. Development of TCI systems	9
	3. Components of a TCI system	11
	4. How do blood-targeted TCI systems deliver steady state blood concentrations?	12
	5. TCI vs Manual infusions	14
II.	**PHARMACOKINETICS**	17
	1. What is a pharmacokinetic model and how is it derived?	17
	2. Pharmacokinetics of commonly used anaesthetic agents	19
	2.1. Propofol	19
	2.2. Remifentanil	20
	2.3. Sufentanil	21
	2.4. Alfentanil	21
	2.5. Fentanyl	21
	2.6. Ketamine	23
	3. Accuracy of target-controlled infusion systems	23
	3.1. Propofol	25
	3.2. Remifentanil	26
	3.3. Sufentanil	26
	3.4. Alfentanil	26
	3.5. Fentanyl	27
	3.6. Ketamine	27
	4. Pharmacokinetic interactions	27
	4.1. Propofol/fentanyl	28
	4.2. Propofol/alfentanil	28
	4.3. Propofol/remifentanil	28
	5. TCI versus manual remifentanil	28
	6. Which figure for patient weight should be used for TIVA and TCI?	30
	7. Effect site targeting, Time to peak effect (TTPE) and k_{eo}	33
	7.1. Effect-site targeting for propofol	37
	7.2. Effect-site targeted opioid infusions	40
III.	**PHARMACODYNAMICS**	43
	1. General	43
	2. Overview of the pharmacodynamics of commonly used anaesthetic agents	43
	2.1. Propofol	43

		2.2. Remifentanil	45
		2.3. Sufentanil	46
		2.4. Alfentanil	46
	3.	Pharmacodynamic interactions	46
IV.	**PRACTICAL ASPECTS**		49
	1.	Manual infusion regimens	49
		1.1. Propofol	49
		1.2. Remifentanil	51
		1.3. Sufentanil	52
		1.4. Ketamine	52
	2.	Induction and maintenance of anaesthesia with TCI propofol	53
		2.1. Blood-targeted TCI	53
		2.2. Effect-site targeted TCI	54
		2.3. Differences between Marsh and Schnider models	55
	3.	Advice for the complete TIVA novice	58
	4.	Target-controlled infusions of opioids	60
	5.	High risk patients (Elderly, unwell, or patients with limited cardiac reserve)	61
	6.	Post-operative analgesia after remifentanil infusions	62
	7.	Combinations of hypnotic and opioid agents	63
		7.1. Propofol and remifentanil	64
		7.2. Inhalational anaesthetic agents and remifentanil	64
	8.	Practical precautions and pitfalls	65
		8.1. Dedicated cannula	65
		8.2. Administration sets	66
		8.3. Single patient use	66
		8.4. Mixing two or more drugs in one syringe	66
		8.5. Drug concentrations	67
		8.6. Concentrated drug solutions, and low target concentrations and/or small patients	68
V.	**THE FUTURE**		69
	1.	New, improved models	69
	2.	New drugs	69
	3.	Patient-controlled TCI systems	70
	4.	Closed loop control of anaesthesia	70
VI.	**CASE STUDIES**		71
	Case 1:	Conscious sedation for insertion of tension-free vaginal tape	71
	Case 2:	Examination under anaesthesia, sigmoidoscopy	74
	Case 3:	Inguinal hernia repair	76

Case 4:	Total hip replacement under combined general and regional anaesthesia (using TCI propofol and epidural local anaesthetic boluses).........	*78*
Case 5:	Clipping of peri-callosal aneurysm using effect-site targeted propofol (Schnider model) and remifentanil infusions (Minto model)	*81*
Case 6:	Excision of skin lesion under general anaesthesia using blood concentration targeted infusions of propofol (Marsh model) and alfentanil (Maitre model)..................................	*84*
Case 7:	Laparotomy for partial bowel resection and reconstruction of ureter ..	*86*

TABLES *89*

REFERENCES.. *95*

General and historical background

WTG Morton performed the first successful public demonstration of anaesthesia in October 1846, when he administered ether by inhalation to Gilbert Abbott at the Massachusetts General Hospital.[1] During the next century anaesthetists continued to induce and maintain anaesthesia almost exclusively via the inhalational route.

Although the idea of injecting drugs intravenously was not new (opium is known to have been injected intravenously in 1665, chloral hydrate in 1872, and chloroform and ether in the early 1900's), intravenous induction of anaesthesia only became common in the 1930's after the discovery of the barbiturates, and intravenous maintenance of anaesthesia has only really become practical, safe and popular in the past decade. Thus intravenous induction and maintenance of anaesthesia has been a relatively recent addition to the anaesthetists' repertoire.

The early intravenous anaesthetic agents such as methohexitone and thiopentone, although suitable for intravenous induction of anaesthesia, are not suitable for use by infusion for maintenance of anaesthesia. In the case of thiopentone accumulation can lead to cardiovascular instability and a very slow recovery, whereas methohexitone is associated with excitatory phenomena and epileptiform changes in the electroencephalogram (EEG). In the decades following the discovery of the barbiturates, ketamine, althesin and etomidate were discovered. Although they possessed desirable pharmacokinetic properties (lack of accumulation), their use was limited by other problems. Ketamine causes excitatory phenomena, nightmares and hallucinations, althesin was associated with a high incidence of anaphylaxis, and prolonged infusions of etomidate were associated with multi-organ failure and death, and even single doses of etomidate have been shown to cause adrenal suppression in critically ill patients.[2]

The discovery of propofol has revolutionised intravenous anaesthesia. First used in 1977, propofol is the only currently available intravenous hypnotic agent suitable for induction and maintenance of anaesthesia.

The discovery, in recent decades, of the shorter-acting opioid analgesics alfentanil and remifentanil, which have a rapid onset and offset of action and are eminently suitable for use by infusion, coupled with technological developments (such as more reliable and accurate intravenous pumps), and advances in our understanding of pharmacokinetic principles have enabled the development of the technique of total intravenous anaesthesia (TIVA) in which anaesthesia is administered exclusively via the intravenous route. Propofol-based TIVA techniques have many advantages. These include rapid recovery of consciousness and psychomotor function, earlier recovery and discharge from the post-anaesthesia care unit[3,4] and shorter times to achieve 'home-readiness'[5] than inhalational anaesthetic techniques. Propofol has an anti-emetic affect[6], and is thus associated with a lower incidence of post-operative nausea and vomiting.[5,7-12] Intravenous agents have no known adverse effects on theatre staff and on the environment.

The ultimate goal, when administering a particular dose of drug, is a specified clinical effect, for which a specific therapeutic concentration at the site of drug action is necessary. This dose-response relationship, summarised in Figure 1, p. 7, can be divided into three parts: the relationship between dose administered and blood concentration (the pharmacokinetic phase), the relationship between effect organ concentration and clinical effect (the pharmacodynamic phase) and the coupling between pharmacokinetics and dynamics. For several decades anaesthetists have been able to control the blood concentration of the inhalational anaesthetic agents by using a vapouriser to administer the drug and by measuring the end-tidal concentration (a reasonable estimate of blood concentration). In this way, anaesthetists who use inhalational anaesthesia need mainly to concern themselves with the pharmacodynamic phase of the dose response relationship.

Until recently, a similar facility to administer stable blood concentrations has not been possible for the intravenous anaesthetic agents. Anaesthetists administering anaesthetic agents via the intravenous route have tended to calculate the dose or infusion rate calculated according to the weight of the patient. The problem with this is the complex relationship between dose and blood and effect-site concentrations. Simple infusion regimens do not yield steady state blood concentration profiles until at least 5 multiples of the elimination half-life. Also, the calculations required to estimate the blood and effect-site concentrations are complex and not amenable to mental arithmetic! While encouraging progress has been made with methods of online estimation of blood propofol concentrations from exhaled gas analysis, these systems require further refinement and development before they could be commercially available.[13,14]

GENERAL AND HISTORICAL BACKGROUND | 7

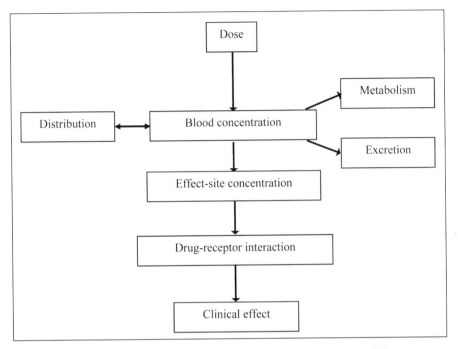

Figure 1: Schematic representation of the pharmacokinetic and dynamic processess determining the relationship between administered dose and resulting clinical effect

I. Target-controlled infusions

1. Definition

A target-controlled infusion is an infusion controlled in such a manner as to attempt to achieve a user-defined drug concentration in a body compartment or tissue of interest. An anaesthetist using a TCI system to administer an anaesthetic agent is thus able to set (and change) a desired concentration (usually referred to as the "target concentration"), based on his clinical observations of the patient. Multi-compartmental pharmacokinetic models, resulting in polyexponential equations, are used by TCI systems to calculate the infusion rates required to achieve the target concentration (see below). A computer or microprocessor is required to perform the complex calculations, and control the infusion pump.

Theoretically, a TCI system can control the concentration in any compartment or tissue in the body. The pharmacokinetic models used are derived from previously performed population pharmacokinetic studies. While a target-controlled infusion is in progress, no measurements of actual concentrations are made, so that these systems are referred to as "open-loop" (as opposed to "closed loop" systems where measurements of the control variable are made, and the errors between the set point and the actual value are used to alter the input to the system). By convention the central compartment in a pharmacokinetic model is referred to as V_c or $V1$, and this compartment includes the vascular compartment. Thus when the target is a user-defined concentration in the central compartment (which includes the vascular compartment), the infusion is called an open-loop blood targeted TCI. When the target concentration is a concentration at the site of action of the drug, the infusion is referred to as an open-loop effect-site targeted TCI.

2. Development of TCI systems

In 1968 Kruger-Thiemer described a theoretical approach to maintaining and achieving a steady state blood concentration of a drug whose pharmacokinetics can be described by a two-compartment model.[15] He showed that in order to achieve steady state blood concentrations it is necessary to administer a loading dose to fill up the initial volume of distribution, an infusion to match the elimination or clearance of the drug load, and a superimposed infusion to match the rate at which the drug is distributed to the peripheral compartment. Vaughan and Tucker[16,17] developed the concept further, as did Schwilden[18] who also developed the first clinical application of this theory, the CATIA system (computer-assisted total intravenous anaesthesia system).

The schemes developed by these pioneers for drugs conforming to a two-compartment model became known as BET (**B**olus, **E**limination, **T**ransfer) schemes. They were called this because they comprised an initial bolus to fill the central compartment, followed by two superimposed infusions, one to replace drug lost by elimination and one to replace drug lost by re-distribution. A fixed proportion of the total amount of drug in the central compartment is eliminated each unit of time. Thus when the blood concentration of a drug is constant the amount of drug eliminated each unit of time is constant, so that drug lost by elimination can be replaced by a constant rate infusion. In contrast the amount of drug distributed to peripheral tissues declines exponentially as the gradient between the central compartment and the peripheral compartment decreases. Thus an infusion at an exponentially declining rate is required to replace drug "lost" from the central compartment by distribution. The sum of these two infusions is naturally an infusion at a decreasing rate.

Since then it has been recognised that the pharmacokinetics of most anaesthetic agents conform best to three-compartment models. Numerous algorithms, appropriate for a three-compartment model, for targeting blood concentrations[19-23] and for targeting effect-site concentrations[24,25] have been published, and several groups of investigators have developed model-driven automated systems capable of delivering steady state drug concentrations. Since the early 1990s the target-controlled infusion software programs developed in Stanford (Stanpump), Stellenbosch (Stelpump) and Gent (RUGLOOP) have been available on request from the authors and are also freely available over the internet (http://anesthesia.stanford.edu/pkpd/). Several pharmacokinetic simulation programs have also been available (examples include IVA-SIM – also available at http://anesthesia.stanford.edu/pkpd/, and TIVATrainer – available at www.eurosiva.org).

Initially, the different groups used different terminology to describe their systems. The best-known terms were: CATIA[18], TIAC (titration of intravenous agents by computer)[26], CACI (computer-assisted continuous infusion)[27], CCIP (computer-controlled infusion pump)[28], and TCI.[29] Eventually a consensus was reached among the leading groups, who published a letter in Anesthesiology suggesting that the term TCI should be adopted.[30] The group also suggested standard nomenclature for blood and effect-site concentrations (C_p and C_e respectively, with the added subscripts T to indicate that the concentration being discussed is the "target" concentration, CALC to indicate that the concentration is the calculated blood or effect-site concentration, and

MEAS to indicate that the blood or effect-site concentration is a measured concentration).

The first commercially available TCI system was the Diprifusor®, a microprocessor that was embedded in intravenous infusion pumps sold by several manufacturers from 1996 onwards (in numerous countries around the world, but not in the USA). The development of the Diprifusor® has been described in detail.[31,32] TCI pumps controlled by it can only administer target-controlled infusions of propofol, and only if the microprocessor is able to detect the presence of single-use pre-filled glass syringes of 1 or 2% propofol purchased from AstraZeneca. These syringes contain a programmable metallic strip in the flange that is detected by a sophisticated process called programmed magnetic resonance. When the syringe is almost empty the strip is "de-programmed" so that it cannot be re-used.

In the years since the release of the first generation of TCI systems, the patent for propofol has expired. While the cost of the pre-filled syringes from Astra-Zeneca has changed very little, significantly cheaper generic forms of propofol are now available. Until recently, propofol purchased from other manufacturers could not be used in TCI propofol systems, but this has now changed with the development and launch of second generation TCI systems, the so-called "Open TCI" systems. These systems allow the use of a variety of drugs, administered from a variety of syringes and sizes. Thus, when used to administer generic propofol formulations, these pumps can generate cost savings of up to 80% of the cost of the original propofol formulation. Two currently available systems are the Alaris Asena PK® (Alaris Medical Systems, Basingstoke, UK), and the Base Primea (Fresenius, Brezins, France).

3.   Components of a TCI system

The basic components of a TCI system are a user interface, a computer or one or more micro-processors and an infusion device. The microprocessor controls the appearance of the user interface, implements the pharmacokinetic model, accepts data input and instructions from the user, performs the necessary mathematical calculations, controls and monitors the infusion device, and implements warning systems to alert the user of any problems (e.g. mains disconnection, syringe almost empty).

Audible and visible warning systems are an essential feature, and TCI devices should be programmed to respond appropriately to all possible fault conditions. Should a serious fault occur, then alarms should sound and the system should shut down or stop infusing, depending on the fault. The first generation TCI pumps contained two microprocessors. A 16-bit microprocessor implemented the algorithm to calculate the infusion rates required for the target concentration, and controlled the syringe driver motor speed accordingly. In parallel, an 8-bit processor monitored the number of rotations of the driving motor and used a simpler mathematical process (involving Euler approximations) to calculate the estimated blood concentration based on the amount of propofol delivered. If the target and estimated blood concentrations differed significantly, the system shut down. As this was a very rare occurrence, the dual processor technique has not been implemented in the new generation pumps.

The user interface prompts and allows the user to enter the patient data such as age, weight, gender and height and of course the target drug concentration, whilst displaying useful numeric and/or graphic information (such as the current infusion rate, and the trend of the calculated blood and effect-site drug concentrations). Typical TCI systems incorporate infusion devices that are capable of infusion rates up to 1200 ml/hr, with a precision of 0.1 ml/hr.

4. How do blood-targeted TCI systems deliver steady state blood concentrations?

TCI systems are programmed with pharmacokinetic models that mathematically describe the processes of drug distribution and elimination (see Figure 2, p. 13, and also the later section on pharmacokinetic models). Although different TCI systems might use slightly different mathematical techniques, the practical end result remains a variation of a BET scheme.

The general method is illustrated in Figure 3, p. 13. When the anaesthetist increases the target concentration the system administers a rapid infusion (bolus) to quickly fill the central compartment thereby giving an almost step-wise increase in blood concentration. The amount infused is calculated according to the estimated central compartment blood volume and the difference between the current calculated and target blood concentrations. When the system calculates that the blood concentration has reached its new target, it stops the rapid infusion, and commences an infusion at a lower rate that is gradually decreasing, to replace drug that is "lost" by distribution and elimination. For practical reasons, current TCI systems repeat the calculations, and alter the infusion rate, at discrete intervals (typically every 10 sec). Thus, although the amount of drug removed from the central compartment changes continuously, the infusion rate used to replace re-distributed and eliminated drug is "step-wise decreasing". If a three-compartment model is used, three superimposed infusions are required. Two first-order exponentially decreasing

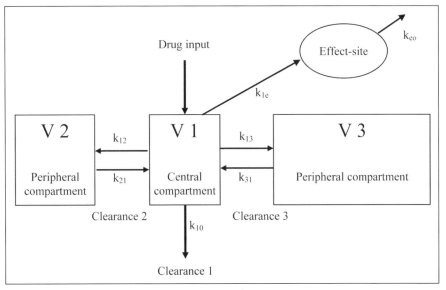

Figure 2: *The three compartment pharmacokinetic model enlarged with an effect compartment. The concentration in this compartment is called "effect-site concentration"*

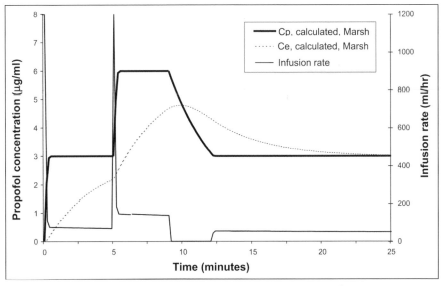

Figure 3: *Blood concentration targeted TCI. At time zero the target is set at 3 µg/ml, at 5 min it is increased to 6 µg/ml., and at 10 min it is reduced to 3 µg/ml. The infusion rates required to achieve these targets are indicated on the right hand vertical axis*

infusions are required to match drug removed from the central compartment to the other two compartments by distribution, while a third infusion (at a constant rate) is required to replace drug removed by elimination.

When the anaesthetist decreases the target concentration the system stops the infusion, and waits until it estimates that the blood concentration has reached the target concentration. The rate at which the blood concentration falls depends on the rate of elimination, and on the gradient between the concentrations in the central and other compartments. Thus if the concentration in the central compartment is greater than that in another compartment, the blood concentration will fall more rapidly, whereas if the reverse is true, the return of drug from the peripheral compartment will reduce the rate of decline in the blood concentration. Once the system estimates the blood concentration has reached the target, it will re-start the infusion at a lower rate, once again calculating the changing infusion rates required to maintain the blood concentration at the target concentration.

5. TCI vs Manual infusions

In most areas of medical practise doctors tend to use manually controlled infusions, usually at a fixed rate. Why is this not sufficient for anaesthesia? The answer lies in the unique requirements of anaesthesia and the pharmacokinetic properties of the anaesthetic drugs. Anaesthesia is one of the few areas of medical practise where it is important to achieve steady state blood and effect-site concentrations, and where it is important for the clinician to be able to exert fine, rapid control over these target concentrations.

When drugs are administered by a fixed rate infusion, the blood concentrations take a very long time to reach a plateau or steady state. This is illustrated for propofol in Figure 4, p. 15, which shows that even after a 12 hour infusion the blood concentrations are still rising. This is because it takes about 24 hours for the drug to equilibrate throughout all the tissues in the body. For drugs such as fentanyl, morphine and midazolam, the time taken for equilibration and steady state is far longer. Thus for the latter drugs and even for propofol large changes to an infusion rate will not lead to significant changes in blood concentration for some time (see Figure 5, p. 15). The time delay before there is a significant change in effect-site concentration, and thus in clinical effect, will be even longer. Excessive concentrations of anaesthetic or analgesic agents may cause adverse effects, whereas with inadequate concentrations the patient is at risk of pain or awareness. These delays are thus generally not acceptable.

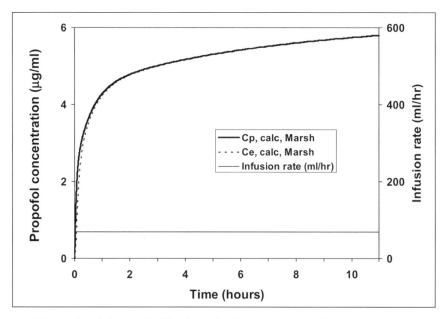

Figure 4: Calculated blood and effect-site propofol concentrations associated with an infusion of 1% propofol at 70 ml/hr for 12 hours in a 70 kg adult

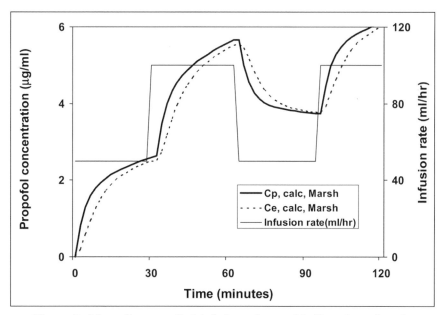

Figure 5: Manually controlled infusion of propofol. Note that when the infusion rate is halved or doubled there is a long delay before the blood propofol concentration halves or doubles

Naturally, when an anaesthetist wants to increase the drug concentration rapidly, he can administer a bolus, but it is difficult to judge the size of bolus appropriate for the patient and the required change. Similarly, if he wants to decrease the concentration as rapidly as possible he can switch off the infusion temporarily, but in the busy theatre environment there is a real risk he may forget to re-start the infusion. With TCI systems, these changes are made automatically, enabling precise and rapid control of the blood concentration.

It is not surprising then that TCI systems are popular with anaesthetists, who have assessed them as easy to use, and providing a high level of predictability of anaesthetic effect.[33] In a study comparing manual infusion with TCI propofol by anaesthetists unfamiliar with propofol infusion anaesthesia, it was found that anaesthetists quickly became familiar with both techniques, but expressed a clear preference for the TCI system.[34]

How does the quality of clinical control compare between TCI and manually controlled infusions? Although many of the early target-controlled infusion systems were used for infusions of opiates, most of the evidence comes from studies comparing TCI with manually controlled propofol infusions. Quality of anaesthesia is difficult to measure, but studies have used simple categorical measures where the anaesthetist rates the quality as good, adequate or poor as well as other numerical methods such as a quality of anaesthesia score.[35] In studies comparing TCI with manual propofol infusion regimens the quality of induction and maintenance of anaesthesia were similar, as was the incidence and severity of haemodynamic effects, and the recovery times.[34,36-40] A large multicentre study found that the control of anaesthesia was easier in subjects anaesthetised with target-controlled than with manually controlled propofol infusions.[41]

II. Pharmacokinetics

Pharmacokinetics is often described as the study of "what the body does to the drug" whereas pharmacodynamics can be described as "what the drug does to the body." In essence pharmacokinetics describes the relationship between the dose administered in mass or molar units, and the resulting blood concentration. TCI devices incorporate a microprocessor programmed with an infusion algorithm that is based on one or more pharmacokinetic models for one or more drugs.

1. What is a pharmacokinetic model and how is it derived?

A pharmacokinetic model is a mathematical model that can be used to predict the blood concentration profile of a drug after a bolus dose or an infusion of varying duration. These models are typically derived by measuring the arterial or venous blood/plasma concentration of a drug after a bolus or infusion, in a group of patients or volunteers, and then using standardised statistical approaches and software such as NONMEM® (a software package for non-linear mixed-effects modelling distributed by Globomax LLC, Hanover, USA) to estimate model parameters in that population.

A 2- or 3-compartment model can be used to mathematically describe the behaviour of most anaesthetic drugs with reasonable accuracy. For most anaesthetic agents in common use there are several published models. Tables 1 (p. 89), 2 (p. 90) and 3 (p. 91) list the model parameters for several commonly used anaesthetic agents. Each model describes the number of compartments, and their volumes, the rate of drug metabolism or elimination, and the rate of transfer of drug between the different compartments. The concept is summarised in Figure 2. By convention the compartment into which the drug is injected is called the central compartment (V1 or Vc). This is also referred to as the initial volume of distribution. The second compartment, V2, is referred to as the "vessel-rich" or "fast re-distribution" compartment (because there is rapid drug distribution between V1 and V2), while the third compartment, V3, is referred to as the "vessel-poor" or "slow" compartment (because there is rather slower drug distribution between V1 and V3). The sum of V1, V2 and V3 gives the "volume of distribution at steady state," Vd_{ss}.

The central compartment may be thought of as including the blood volume, but note that V1 may be far larger than the blood volume (see Table 1, p. 89). It is important to remember that the "volumes" of a 2- or 3-compartment model are theoretical volumes that can be used to predict blood concentrations – they have no real anatomical or physiological correlates.

The rates of drug metabolism and distribution can be interchangeably described by rate constants or clearances. A rate constant describes a proportion of drug in a compartment undergoing a process during a unit of time, and is thus reported with the units min^{-1} or hr^{-1}. By convention we use the symbol k_{10} to denote the rate constant for metabolism or elimination, whereas the symbols k_{12}, k_{21}, k_{13} and k_{31} are used to denote the rate constants for drug transfer between V1 and V2, between V2 and V1, between V1 and V3, and between V3 and V1 respectively.

A brief example seeking to explain rate constants follows. If for drug X, the rate constants k_{13} and k_{31} are 0.05 and 0.005 respectively, this means that in each unit of time 5% of the total amount of drug X in compartment 1 moves into compartment 3, whereas 0.5% of the amount of drug X in compartment 3 moves into compartment 1 in each unit of time. Clearly the nett movement of drug X, in mass or molar units, depends on the relative concentrations of drug X in the two compartments. If, for example, compartment 1 has a volume of 10 litres and the concentration of drug X at time zero is 1 µg/ml, then the amount of drug moving from compartment 1 to compartment 3 in the next minute is 500 µg (5% × 1 µg/ml × 10,000 ml). As can be seen below it follows from the ratio of the rate constants that the volume of compartment 3 must be 100 litres (10 litres × 0.05/0.005). If the concentration in this compartment happens to be 0.1 µg/ml at time zero, then the amount of drug moving from compartment 3 to compartment 1 is 50 µg (0.5% of 10,000 µg) and so the nett result is an overall increase in the amount of drug X in compartment 3 of 450 µg.

Clearances on the other hand describe a volume (of a compartment) that is "cleared" during a unit of time. The units are thus ml/min or ml/hr. If the compartment volume and the rate constants are known the clearances are easily calculated as follows:

Elimination clearance $= V1 \times k_{10}$

Clearance 2 $= V2 \times k_{21}$

Clearance 3 $= V3 \times k_{31}$

Sometimes when models are reported in the literature, only V1 and the various rate constants are listed. This is because V2 and V3 can be deduced from the rate constants as follows:

$$V2 = V1 \times \frac{k_{12}}{k_{21}}$$

$$V3 = V1 \times \frac{k_{13}}{k_{31}}$$

2. Pharmacokinetics of commonly used anaesthetic agents

2.1. Propofol

2.1.1. Adults

The pharmacokinetic model with which most anaesthetists are familiar is the three compartment model published by Marsh at al.[42] It is incorporated in the Diprifusor® (AstraZeneca, Macclesfield, UK), a microprocessor that until recently was used in all commercially available TCI pumps. This model was an adaptation of that originally published by Gepts et al.[43] In this model the central compartment volume is a linear function of the weight of the patient, while the rate constants are fixed. Although the Diprifusor software also requires the user to enter an age for each patient, the model described by Marsh et al does not incorporate age as a co-variate (the system will not function if an age < 16 is entered).

Since then several studies have demonstrated that age, gender, height, mode of administration (bolus versus infusion) and site of blood sampling (venous vs. arterial) all influence the pharmacokinetic model parameters. Schüttler et al analysed the data from several studies of propofol pharmacokinetics in adults and children and produced a model that incorporates all the aforementioned factors and is valid for patients of all ages.[44] In his model all parameters except for V3 are derived from equations that include a power function of body weight. Elimination clearance and V1 are also influenced by age. Schnider et al developed a model that includes a fixed V1, with age as a co-variate in the calculation of V2 and Clearance2, and weight, height and lean body mass as co-variates for the metabolic (elimination) clearance.[45] Table 1, p. 89, lists the parameters for these adult propofol models for a male who is 40 years old, 170 cm tall and weighs 70 kg.

2.1.2. Children

During the early 1990s the accuracy of target-controlled infusions using the Marsh model in 20 children was studied, and found to be associated with a significant over-estimation in the blood concentrations (i.e. measured blood concentrations were less than expected).[42] This was consistent with the findings of several groups of workers who have found that the pharmacokinetics of propofol differ between children and adults.[46,47] The Marsh model was then revised to produce a model specific to children (the size of the central compartment volume was increased, but remained a linear function of body weight), and when prospectively tested, the predictive performance was better than when the adult model was used.[42] Since then several other models specific to children have been produced.

Two models are commonly used at present. Kataria et al developed a three compartmental model for propofol in children using three different pharmacokinetic modelling techniques in an extended group of children between 3 and 11 years.[48] This model has fixed rate constants, while compartmental volumes have a linear correlation with weight. The Paedfusor model[49] was adapted from one of the preliminary models developed by Schüttler prior to the publication of his final model,[44] and was incorporated in a paediatric TCI pump developed and used in Glasgow. In the Paedfusor model the central compartment volume and clearance have a non-linear correlation with weight, whereas in the final Schüttler model all variables have a non-linear correlation with age and weight. Table 2, p. 90, shows the models, along with parameters for a representative child (weight 20kg) for the Paedfusor and Kataria models. Another model specific to children is the Short[50] model but this is seldom used.

2.2. Remifentanil

Remifentanil is a newer synthetic opioid that is ultra- short-acting owing to the fact that it is metabolised by non-specific esterases present in most tissues of the body. Whereas most other anaesthetic agents need to be present in the blood, and then to pass through the hepatic circulation before they can be inactivated by hepatic metabolism, remifentanil is metabolised wherever it is in the body. Remifentanil pharmacokinetics are thus not modified by hepatic[51] or renal failure.[52]

The model most commonly used for remifentanil is a 3-compartment model described by Minto.[53,54] This model was produced from a study of the pharmacokinetics of remifentanil in a heterogeneous population (there was wide variation in age and body weight). Co-variates include weight, height and gender (from which lean body mass are calculated), and age. The model parameters for a 40 yr old male who weighs 70 kg can be seen in Table 3, p. 91.

Note the small sizes of the compartments and the relatively large rate constants for metabolism and re-distribution.

2.3. Sufentanil

Sufentanil is a potent synthetic opioid whose pharmacokinetics are best described by a three compartment model. Commonly used models include those developed by Gepts[55] and Bovill[56] (see Table 3, p. 91). Both models are characterised by a large volume of distribution (V3 is particularly large) and a high metabolic clearance. Because of the large V3, the terminal half-life of sufentanil is long. In the model described by Bovill et al, V1 is a linear function of body weight while the rate constants are fixed,[56] whereas in the model described by Gepts et al the volumes of the compartments are fixed (i.e. not adjusted for weight) as are the rate constants.[55] Age does not appear to influence the pharmacokinetics of sufentanil.[57]

2.4. Alfentanil

Alfentanil is approximately 10 times more potent than morphine but is less fat-soluble than many other anaesthetic drugs. It is metabolised in the liver, but has a relatively low extraction ratio of 0.3-0.5.[58-60] Various compartmental models for alfentanil were developed in the early 1980's.[58,59,61,62] The major drawback from all these original studies was the lack of formal population modelling approach. Maitre used the original datasets from the 4 above mentioned studies and developed a new model using non linear mixed-effect modeling (NONMEM)[63]. His three compartmental model has been found to be accurate and is the most commonly used model for TCI alfentanil systems. It incorporates weight, age and gender as co-variables in the calculation of compartment volumes and elimination and distribution rate constants. As a consequence of the pharmacokinetic characteristics of alfentanil the model is characterised by small compartmental volumes, and a relatively small elimination rate constant (Table 3, p. 91).

2.5. Fentanyl

The potency of fentanyl is approximately 100-fold more potent than morphine, reflecting it's greater lipid solubility. Onset of action shorter than with morphine, but similar to that of alfentanil while the duration of action is longer than alfentanil, but shorted than morphine. Despite the clinical impression that fentanyl produces a rapid onset, the time to peak effect is ~3.5 minutes, because of the rather slow equilibration time between blood and the brain for fentanyl. Fentanyl has a large volume of distribution. The relatively short duration of action of a single dose reflects its rapid redistribution to inactive tissue sites such as fat and skeletal muscles, with an associated decrease in the plasma concentration of the drug. The lungs also serve as a large, inactive storage site, with an estimated 75% of the initial fentanyl close undergoing first-pass pulmonary uptake.[64] This non-respiratory function of the lungs limits the initial amount of drug that reaches the systemic circulation and may play an important role in determining the pharmacokinetic profile of fentanyl.

Fentanyl undergoes extensive hepatic metabolism, producing inactive metabolites. Less than 10% is excreted unchanged in the urine. It is a substrate for hepatic P-450 enzymes (CYP3A) and so is susceptible to interactions with drugs that influence enzyme activity.

When repeated doses or infusions of fentanyl are administered, the context-sensitive half-time increases dramatically as the duration of administration increases, becoming longer than that of sufentanil after 2 hours (see the section on Context-Sensitive Half-Time).[65,66]

The pharmacokinetics of fentanyl are best described by a three compartment model. The first models for fentanyl were produced by McClain,[67] Hudson[68] and Scott[69]. The McClain and Scott models were later assessed by Shafer who tested their predictive performance during computer controlled fentanyl infusions. Shafer found that the MDAPE for the McClain model was 61% whereas the MDAPE for the Scott model was 33%,[28] and went on to use a pooled data approach to produce a new model which performed well when used to (retrospectively) predict fentanyl concentrations in the 21 patients in his study, as well as the concentrations in 4 previous studies. This model is thus commonly used for TCI fentanyl administration.

In common with the other models mentioned above, the Shafer model has no covariates, and this is reasonable when applied to a population of patients similar to those in whom the model was developed (a group of non-obese patients). Shibutani recently studied the predictive performance of the Shafer model in lean and obese patients.[70] While the model performed reasonably well in lean patients, in the obese it systematically overpredicted blood concentrations as total body mass increased. Thus, if infusions are used, methods of improving predictive accuracy include use of a "pharmacokinetic mass" or "dosing mass" calculated from total body weight, or an adjustment factor applied to the target concentration.

2.6. Ketamine

Except in circumstances such as in battlefield anaesthesia, repeated procedures for burns, and anaesthesia in developing countries, ketamine is seldom used as the sole hypnotic agent because of the adverse emergence phenomena. Recently there has been a resurgence of interest in this drug because of growing evidence that surgical patients may benefit from low-dose intraoperative infusions. Potential benefits include neuroprotection,[71] pre-emptive analgesia and attenuation of post-operative hyperalgesia.[72] The influence of low-dose ketamine on postoperative analgesia was the subject of a recent Cochrane review.[73] Target-controlled infusion technology has been employed for ketamine administration in several settings, including critical care,[74,75] the operating theatre,[76-78] and neuroscience studies.[79,80] At Cambridge University, ketamine infusions are being used to investigate the glutaminergic hypofunction theory of schizophrenia.[81-87]

Several models have been produced for ketamine, mostly from studies involving small numbers of patients. Most of the models have 3 compartments[88-91] although the Clements model[92] and a model published recently by Hijazi[75] have only two. The three compartment Domino model[89] (see Table 3, p. 91) is the most commonly used model for TCI ketamine administration.

3. Accuracy of target-controlled infusion systems

A TCI system administers a drug infusion regimen at rates determined by a model derived from studies of the pharmacokinetics of that drug in a population of patients or subjects. It is important to remember that the concentration shown on the user interface is only an estimate. At present there is no method of measuring the actual drug concentration in real time, analogous to the infrared end-tidal volatile anaesthetic analyser found on most anaesthetic machines, which gives the reassurance that the drug is at least reaching the patient.

Many factors can influence the actual drug concentrations achieved. Thanks to technological developments and strict regulatory controls, technical factors (such as the accuracy of the motors that drive infusion pumps and correct microprocessor programming to ensure proper implementation of pharmacokinetic models) are unlikely to be significant. More relevant factors are whether or not the drug is actually reaching the intravascular space (there may be a line disconnection or the intravenous cannula may not be in a vein) and whether or not the pharmacokinetic model applies to a specific patient.

Fortunately, offline retrospective analysis of blood samples is possible, and numerous studies have thus been performed to assess the predictive accuracy of the pharmacokinetic models in various groups of subjects. In 1992 Varvel and colleagues proposed a set of standard criteria for assessing the predictive performance of computerised infusion pumps.[93] These criteria are MDPE (median performance error, a measure of bias or offset), MDAPE (median absolute performance error, a measure of inaccuracy or imprecision), wobble (a measure of the intra-individual variability in errors) and divergence (a measure of any trend over time in the size and magnitude of errors). To calculate these criteria it is necessary to first calculate the performance error (PE) for each measured drug concentration, C_{meas}, where the calculated or predicted concentration is C_{pred}, as follows:

For the jth measurement in the ith patient:

$$PE_{ij} = \frac{(C_{meas} - C_{pred})}{C_{pred}} \times 100$$

The four criteria are then calculated as follows:

For the ith patient for whom N_i drug assays were performed

$MDPE_i = \text{Median } \{PE_{ij}, j = 1, ..., N_i\}$

$MDAPE_i = \text{Median } \{|PE_{ij}|, j = 1, ..., N_i\}$

$Wobble_i = \text{Median } \{|PE_{ij} - MDPE_i|, j = 1, ..., N_i\}$

Divergence: is calculated for each individual as the slope of the linear regression of that individual's absolute performance errors over time (a positive value indicates that the performance errors are increasing over time, whereas a negative value indicates that the measured values are converging with the predicted values over time)

For computer-controlled infusion pumps a MDPE (bias) of 10-20% and a MDAPE of 20-40% have been proposed as acceptable.[94,95] These figures can be put into perspective when one considers the "accuracy" of end-tidal volatile agent monitoring. The output from the anaesthetic vapouriser is usually accurate to within a few percent of that indicated on the dial. Standard teaching holds that if the measured end-tidal concentration and the atmospheric pressure are known, one can calculate the end-tidal partial pressure, and that this is the same as the arterial tension of the anaesthetic agent in question. However, studies comparing the end-tidal and measured arterial concentrations of isoflurane have shown that end-tidal concentrations under-predict arterial concentrations by 20%.[96,97]

So how well do the different pharmacokinetic models match up to these standards? A full discussion of the performance of all the models for the drugs mentioned above is beyond the scope of this booklet. Naturally the best performing models tend to be the ones most commonly used. In the following section the performance of the "better" models will be highlighted. A summary of the information is given in Table 4, p. 92.

3.1. Propofol

3.1.1. Adults

The two main models in use are those described by Marsh[42] and Schnider[45]. No formal studies of the predictive performance of the Schnider model have been published.

The publication in which the Marsh model parameters were first presented did not include the results of a validation study of the model in adults. The paper was actually a report of a study of the performance of the model in children, followed by the results of a prospective study of a new model specific for children (developed from retrospective analysis of the data from the earlier study). Since then several studies of the predictive performance of the Marsh model have been performed (some are highlighted in Table 4). Most tend to show that the Marsh model under-predicts the blood concentration (positive bias). An exception was the study performed by Coetzee et al that showed a MDPE of –7% and a MDAPE of 18%.[98] A study of the 'Diprifusor' in adult general surgical patients found an overall MDPE of 16% and an overall MDAPE of 24%.[99] In another study in patients undergoing cardiac surgery the MDPE was 23% and the MDAPE 19% (both figures before bypass).[100] Davidson et al found similar results in patients undergoing breast surgery, but also interestingly found that the predictive performance was better when the infusion device was not actively infusing propofol (such as after a reduction in target concentration) than when it was infusing propofol (MDPE improved from 21.4% to –2%, and MDAPE improved from 30.2% to 15.1%).[101]

Most studies of the Marsh model have included young and middle-aged patients. An exception was the study by Swinhoe et al, which included 68 patients with ages between 56 and 80.[99] Although the median MDPE and MDAPE values were similar for the younger and older age groups, there was a broader range of values found in the older age group (for one patient the MDPE and MDAPE were 84%!). Because the Schnider model uses age and

LBM as co-variates, it may be a safer model to use when administering propofol to elderly patients.

3.1.2. Children

Studies of the predictive performance of the Marsh model in children have shown that it over-predicts blood concentrations (bias is of the order of –20%, meaning that measured concentrations tend to be 20% lower than those calculated by the system).[42-50] The revised Marsh (paediatric) model showed a far better bias,[49] as did the Short model which showed bias of –0.1% and precision of 21.5%.[50] The Paedfusor model performed very well when it was studied in 29 children undergoing cardiac surgery or cardiac catheterisation – bias was 4.1% and precision 9.7% (Table 4, p. 92).[49] There are no peer-reviewed publications of prospective studies of the predictive performance of the Kataria model.

3.2. Remifentanil

Mertens and colleagues studied the predictive performance of several remifentanil models during propofol/remifentanil anaesthesia.[102] For the Minto model they found a bias of –15% and precision of 20%. Drover et al studied the predictive performance of the Minto model in 40 patients undergoing abdominal surgery and found a similar precision (18.2%), but a much better bias of 1.59%.

3.3. Sufentanil

Studies of the predictive performance of the Gepts model show acceptable bias and precision. Most of the studies have shown a tendency for the Gepts model to overpredict the blood concentration (i.e. MDPE or bias negative). Barvais et al found values of –22.3 and 29.0%,[103] Pandin et al found values of –10.0 and 20.7%,[104] and Hudson found values of –2.3 and 20.7% respectively.[105] Slepchenko et al studied sufentanil pharmacokinetics in obese patients, and found that with the Gepts model (in which compartment volumes and rate constants are not weight-adjusted) the performance indices were similar (bias –12.8% and precision 19.8%).[106]

3.4. Alfentanil

Maitre et al tested the predictive performance of his model in adult patients undergoing abdominal and superficial surgery, and found acceptable results: MDPE was –7.9 and MDAPE 22.3%.[107] However, when Barvais et al studied several alfentanil models in elderly patients he found that the Maitre model tended to underpredict the blood alfentanil concentration (i.e. bias or MDPE were positive) and the inaccuracy (MDAPE) was > 40%.[108]

3.5. Fentanyl

As mentioned previously Shafer found that the MDAPE for the McClain model was 61% whereas the MDAPE for the Scott model was 33%.[28] Shibutani and colleagues studied the predictive performance of the Shafer model in lean and obese patients,[70] and found that while the model performed reasonably well in lean patients, in the obese it systematically overpredicted blood concentrations as total body mass increased. The authors examined various solutions to this problem, and recommended that clinicians who wish to use TCI fentanyl use the Shafer model as it is (none of the parameters are weight-adjusted), but make a fairly simple upward adjustment to the target concentration in the obese.[70]

3.6. Ketamine

In a retrospective study of the predictive performance of the Domino model during 4 studies involving low-dose target-controlled ketamine infusions, performance was sub-optimal.[109] The model significantly overpredicted ketamine blood concentrations for the first hour of infusion, and then after a further hour or so, and particularly after the infusion were stopped, it tended to underpredict ketamine concentrations. A new pharmacokinetic model has been developed and is undergoing prospective evaluation in Cambridge.

4. Pharmacokinetic interactions

Pharmacokinetic interactions occur when the presence of one drug causes an alteration in the pharmacokinetics of another agent. They are common among anaesthetic agents, of which the interactions between propofol and various opioid agents are described in most detail. Proposed mechanisms for these interactions include competition between propofol and opioids for pulmonary binding sites,[110] inhibition by propofol of cytochrome P450,[111] and haemodynamic alterations caused by propofol.[112] It is also likely that at higher concentrations propofol alters its own metabolism by causing changes to cardiac output and hepatic blood flow.

When combinations of drugs are used the blood concentrations are slightly higher than expected – of the order of 15-40% greater (see below). While these interactions should be borne in mind, it is seldom necessary to alter the target concentrations used because of pharmacokinetic interactions. In contrast, the synergism arising from pharmacodynamic interactions among anaesthetic agents is of greater significance and commonly requires a decrease of target concentration.

4.1. Propofol/fentanyl

Cockshott et al found that if 100 µg of fentanyl is given before a bolus of propofol, the subsequent propofol concentrations are 50% greater than expected.[113]

4.2. Propofol/alfentanil

Pavlin et al, when comparing propofol concentrations in subjects receiving propofol alone with those in subjects receiving both propofol and alfentanil infusions, found that a target alfentanil concentration of 40ng/ml was associated with a 19-29% increase in propofol concentration.[114] In the same study, *alfentanil* concentrations were also significantly higher when it was infused with propofol than when it was infused alone.

Mertens and colleagues studied the pharmacokinetics of propofol in male volunteers and found significant reductions in elimination clearance (metabolism) and in inter-compartmental clearance rates for alfentanil in the presence of propofol.[112]

4.3. Propofol/remifentanil

Bouillon and colleagues have shown that co-administration of propofol with remifentanil causes 41% decreases in the central compartment volume and distributional clearance, and a 15% decrease in the elimination clearance of remifentanil.[115] Remifentanil did not appear to alter the pharmacokinetics of propofol.

5. TCI versus manual remifentanil

When fixed rate remifentanil infusions are used steady state concentrations are reached far sooner than with most other anaesthetic drugs (after an infusion duration of about 20 minutes the blood concentrations reach a plateau). More importantly, the decline in remifentanil concentration after an infusion is stopped is far more predictable than the decline found with other drugs. Regardless of the duration of the infusion the context-sensitive half-time (the time after the infusion is stopped that it takes for the blood concentration to fall by 50%) remains of the order of 4 minutes. This context-insensitivity is in stark contrast with most other anaesthetic agents whose context-sensitive half-times increase with the duration of the infusion.[66,116]

These beneficial pharmacokinetic properties of remifentanil have led many to question the need for TCI remifentanil systems. Many anaesthetists administer manually controlled remifentanil infusions using fairly simple regimens in which the infusion rate is calculated only on the basis of the weight of the patient. While weight-adjusted infusion regimens work well for young healthy patients they can give far higher blood concentrations than expected in elderly or unwell patients. The simulation in Figure 6 uses the Minto model to show the predicted blood concentrations that would arise from the same infusion profile in two female patients both weighing 60 kg, but with different heights and weights. In both remifentanil is infused at 0.5 µg/kg/min for 3 min and thereafter at 0.25 µg/kg/min. After 15 min the blood concentration in the younger, taller patient is approximately 5 ng/ml, whereas in the older, shorter patient the blood concentration is about 8 ng/ml. Given that the elderly patient is likely to also have greater (pharmacodynamic) sensitivity to the effects of remifentanil, this concentration is likely to result in clinical effects at least twice as great as those in the younger patient, with the potential for serious adverse effects.

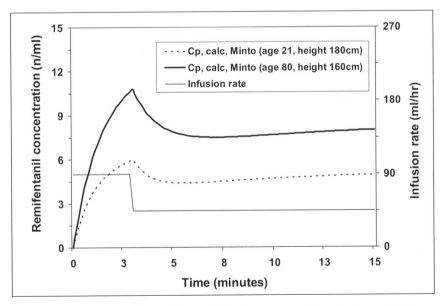

Figure 6: Estimated remifentanil blood concentrations during weight-adjusted manual infusions in two female patients who both weigh 60 kg, but have different heights and ages. Note that in the older, shorter patient far higher blood concentrations arise than in the younger, taller patient

Thus while manual infusion regimens are probably satisfactory in younger, fitter patients in whom excessive concentrations are better tolerated, in the elderly and unwell more precise administration regimens are required. Minto found that the pharmacokinetics of remifentanil are affected by age, gender and height, in addition to weight. It would be too time-consuming and complicated for an anaesthetist to calculate infusion rates based on all these co-variables (even with a calculator). One solution for anaesthetists administering remifentanil to elderly patients is to make an arbitrary adjustment in the weight-adjusted dose, but this is a fairly crude solution. The most precise control of remifentanil concentrations can be achieved with a TCI system that is programmed with a sophisticated model (e.g. Minto) that adjusts for all known co-variables.

6. Which figure for patient weight should be used for TIVA and TCI?

For most drugs used in clinical practise, whether by bolus or infusion or both, the doses and infusion rates recommended in the package inserts are calculated on a weight-adjusted basis. The problem with this is that most of the pharmacokinetic studies involving anaesthetic agents have only included healthy, non-obese patients, and very few have specifically studied the pharmacokinetic properties of these drugs in obese patients. While the recommended weight-adjusted doses apply to most patients, anaesthetists in clinical practise soon intuitively realise that they do not apply to obese, elderly or unwell patients, for whom a smaller dose will usually be given. For example, a patient who is 170 cm tall and weighs 160 kg does not usually need twice as much propofol to induce anaesthesia as a patient who has the same height but weighs only 80 kg. Conversely, two patients of similar weight, but with marked differences in height and age, do not require the same dose of remifentanil (Figure 6) to achieve the same blood concentration.

The intuitive inclination of anaesthetists to reduce the weight-adjusted dose in the obese is supported by studies that have shown a good correlation between dose requirements and **lean body mass** for propofol[117], thiopentone,[118] and atracurium.[119] A study by Egan and colleagues of remifentanil pharmacokinetics in obese and non-obese patients showed that if doses are calculated according to total body weight, then measured concentrations are significantly higher in obese patients.[120] Also the study showed that if compartment volumes are clearances are adjusted for lean body mass, then the pharmacokinetics among obese and non-obese patients are similar, leading the authors to conclude that dose regimens for remifentanil should be based on ideal body weight or lean body mass.

When a drug is administered as a target-controlled infusion (i.e. by a microprocessor controlled infusion pump) the choice of which figure to use for patient weight is even more critical, because the pump uses a model that makes assumptions about clearance rates and volumes of distribution that will have a significant impact on ongoing infusion rates and the total dose administered. Older models used for target-controlled infusions, use total body weight to calculate either or both of V1 and metabolic clearance. One example is the Marsh model, and so when using this model to administer propofol to obese patients, anaesthetists experienced in intravenous anaesthesia will tend to input into the pump a lower value than the measured total body weight. One strategy is to have an arbitrary maximum weight, and if the patient weighs more than that, input that maximum value. It is important to remember, of course, that the maximum value used should depend on the height of the patient. A very tall patient who is very heavy may not be obese! Another strategy is to estimate the patient's ideal body weight and then to use a figure somewhere between the ideal weight and the measured total body weight. A commonly used method of calculating ideal body weight is by using the following formulae[121]:

Males: Ideal body weight (kg) = 49.9 + 0.89 × (height in cm - 152.4)
Females: Ideal body weight (kg) = 45.4 + 0.89 × (height in cm - 152.4)

More recent models, such as those published by Schnider and colleagues for propofol, and by Minto and colleagues for remifentanil, are more complex and use age and **lean body mass** (LBM) as co-variables. These models require the user to enter the total body weight, height and gender, and then use these variables to calculate the lean body mass according to the following formulae[122]:

Males: LBM = 1.1 × weight − 128 × (weight/height)^2
Females: LBM = 1.07 × weight − 148 × (weight/height)^2

At first glance the use of LBM may seem like a sensible idea, and so it is for the non-obese population, for whom the equations give a reasonable approximation of the ideal body mass (Figure 7). The problem is that these equations do not apply to the (growing) population of extremely obese patients. As can be seen from the equations, for a given height, as the weight increases the LBM will increase, but a threshold will be reached beyond which the LBM will decrease (which is counter-intuitive) and eventually become negative (which is absurd)! This is illustrated in Figure 7, p. 32.

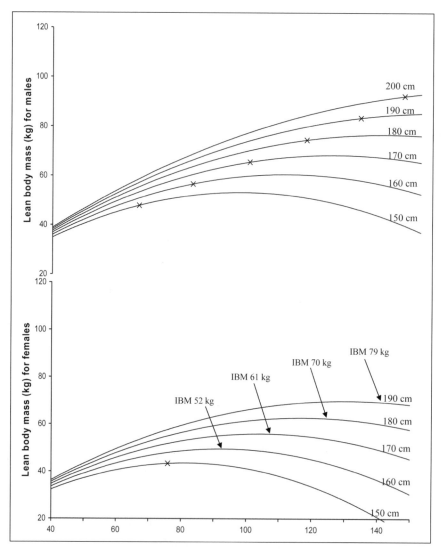

Figure 7: Relationship between body weight, height, lean and ideal body weight (LBM and IBW) for males (top panel) and females (lower panel). Each line shows the change in LBM for a given height (indicated on the right). IBWs for each height are indicated by crosses or text and arrows (when the IBW does not fall on the LBM curve)

Automated infusion systems that seek to implement the Schnider and Minto models (and indeed any other model using LBM), should be programmed with a strategy for dealing with extremely obese patients. A system that blindly uses the LBM formulae given above for an extremely obese patient, is likely to administer far too little drug! One approach is for the microprocessor to be programmed with absolute weight limits for total body weight, and to simply refuse to operate in TCI mode when those limits are exceeded. A more sophisticated approach is to program the pump to refuse to operate in TCI mode if the total weight exceeds the weight that generates the maximum LBM from the equations. In this situation the best compromise is probably to program the pump to suggest that the user inputs the body weight that generates the maximum LBM. For example if the patient is female and 150 cm tall but weighs more than 80 kg (see Figure 7), the pump should either refuse to operate in TCI mode, or suggest that the user inputs a value of 80 kg. It will be important for him to bear in mind though, that while this will cause the pump to infuse a larger dose than it would have if the equation had been blindly followed, the mass of drug required to achieve any given target concentration is likely to be greater for this patient (who weighs more than 80 kg) than it is for a patient of similar height who weighs 80 kg.

Given these complications and difficulties, it is important that an anaesthetist who wishes to administer a target-controlled infusion with a system that uses LBM should be aware of how that system deals with the problem of extreme obesity, and make appropriate allowances and adjustments if necessary.

7. Effect site targeting, Time to peak effect (TTPE) and k_{eo}

First generation TCI systems incorporated the Diprifusor micro-processor, which is programmed to target the blood concentration. Although some models were able to display the calculated effect-site concentration, they were unable to directly target the effect-site concentration. The problem with targeting the blood concentration is that when the target concentration is changed there is a temporal delay before the concentration at the effect-site equilibrates with the blood concentration. As the clinical effect of a drug depends on the concentration at the effect-site, there is usually a hysteresis in clinical effect when the target blood concentration of the agent is increased and then decreased. In fact it was, in part, the observation made by anaesthetists using early propofol TCI systems that patients lost and regained consciousness at different estimated blood concentrations that lead to the realisation that blood-effect-site equilibration is not instantaneous; and that when blood concentrations were changing it was the effect-site (and not the blood) concentration that determined the clinical effect.

The rate of equilibration between blood and effect-site depends on several factors. These include the factors that influence the rate of delivery of the drug to the effect-site (such as cardiac output and cerebral blood flow) and the pharmacological properties of the drug that determine the rate of transfer of the drug across the blood-brain barrier (lipid solubility, degree of ionisation etc). The time course of blood-effect-site equilibration can be mathematically described by a rate constant typically referred to as the k_{eo}. Strictly speaking k_{eo} should be used to describe the rate of removal of drug from the effect-site out of the body, but the effect-site is usually regarded as a volume-less additional compartment, so that there is no need for separate constants describing the rate constants for movement into *and out of* the effect compartment.

Naturally the concentration at the effect-site cannot be directly measured, and most of the time the blood concentration is not known either. However, the time-course of the changes in the effect-site concentration can be estimated from measures of clinical (pharmacodynamic) effect such as spontaneous or evoked EEG parameters. When the blood concentration in a group of subjects is known then pharmacodynamic measures can be used to estimate the k_{eo}, the rate constant used to mathematically describe the time course of equilibration between the blood and effect-site in those subjects, and the combined pharmacokinetic-pharmacodynamic model may be applicable to a similar population.

When pharmacodynamic and pharmacokinetic data are not available from the same subject group then it is recommended that the time to peak effect (TTPE), a model-independent parameter, is be used to estimate the k_{eo} for a pharmacokinetic model and patient group.[102] For a given patient, and a given drug, bolus administration of a drug will result in a rapid increase in blood concentration, followed by a bi- or tri-exponential decline, the rate of which is determined by the rates of drug distribution and metabolism. The rate of change of drug concentration in the compartments is determined by the concentration gradient between the central and other compartments, and by the inter-compartmental drug distribution rate constants. Thus the time-course of changes in the effect-site is determined by the blood-effect-site concentration gradient. When the blood concentration is greater than the concentration in the effect-site, the effect-site concentration rises, and vice versa. After a bolus the maximum effect-site drug concentration occurs at the point when the blood and effect-site concentration curves cross (see Figure 8, p. 35). As the clinical effect is determined by the effect-site concentration, the time delay between a bolus injection and the time at which the blood and effect-site concentration curves cross or intersect, is referred to as the "time to peak effect" (TTPE). It is important to remember that in general, the time to peak effect of a given drug in a given patient is independent of the size of the bolus dose.

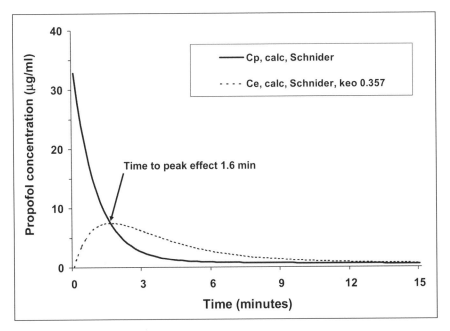

Figure 8: Calculated blood and effect-site propofol concentrations after a 2 mg/kg propofol bolus is administered to an 18 year old male, who weighs 70 kg and is 160 cm tall. A k_{eo} of 0.357 min^{-1} results in a TTPE of 1.6 min

If the same bolus dose (calculated on a mg/kg basis) is administered to two different patients then simpler models such as the Marsh model for propofol will predict the same peak blood concentration, and the same time-course of blood drug concentration. In this case, the same TTPE will generate the same k_{eo} for all patients. When more complex multi-variate models are used (e.g. Schnider, Minto) they tend to predict different peaks and time-courses of blood concentrations for patients with different characteristics. When a more complex pharmacokinetic model is used, and the TTPE for that drug and population is known, then that TTPE can be used to calculate a unique k_{eo} for each patient.

With a blood-targeted TCI system, the user defines the blood concentration, and the effect-site concentration follows passively, with a time delay determined by the k_{eo} or TTPE for the drug in use. When the k_{eo} is used in conjunction with the pharmacokinetic parameters, it is possible to "target" the effect-site rather than the blood concentration. With effect-site targeting the system manipulates the blood concentration to bring about the target (effect-site) concentration as rapidly as possible. This is illustrated in Figure 9, p. 36. When the target effect-site concentration is increased the system calculates an optimal peak blood concentration that will cause a gradient sufficient to cause the most rapid increase in effect-site concentration but without an overshoot of the targeted effect-site concentration. Once the system estimates that this calculated blood concentration has been reached the infusion is switched off. If the peak was calculated correctly the (declining) blood and (increasing) effect-site concentrations will reach the target simultaneously. The system will then re-start the infusion to maintain the blood (and effect-site) concentrations at the target concentration.

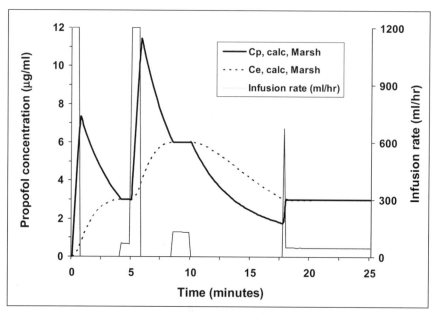

Figure 9: Effect-site targeted TCI. At time zero the target is set at 3 µg/ml, at 5 min it is increased to 6 µg/ml., and at 10 min it is reduced to 3 µg/ml. At each target change the system manipulates the blood concentration to rapidly achieve the target effect-site concentration

If the target effect-site concentration is decreased the system switches off the infusion, and allows the blood concentration to fall below the target level, thereby creating a gradient driving drug out of the effect-site. This causes the most rapid possible decline in effect-site concentration. As soon as the effect-site concentration reaches the target, the infusion is re-started. A bolus is given, followed by an infusion to maintain the blood and effect-site concentrations at the target concentration.

Anaesthetists planning to use an effect-site targeted system need to bear in mind the fact that there are layers of assumptions inherent in effect-site targeting. Pharmacokinetic parameters and models, based on population studies, may not apply to an individual, and measured blood concentrations may be quite different to those predicted. The choice of k_{eo} value used is especially critical in effect-site targeting, because it will determine the overshoot and undershoot in blood concentrations used to steer the effect-site concentration when the target effect-site concentration is increased or decreased respectively. If two different systems use the same pharmacokinetic data set, but with different k_{eo} values, different drug doses will be administered leading to different peak and trough blood concentrations. A "slower" k_{eo} value (i.e. a smaller rate constant) will cause a higher peak blood concentration when the target concentration is increased and a deeper trough when the target is decreased.

In summary it is very important that a fixed k_{eo} should only be used for effect-site targeting when both kinetic and dynamic models have been calculated from the same study population. If this is not possible, then a time to peak effect algorithm should be used.

7.1. *Effect-site targeting for propofol*

7.1.1. *Effect-site targeting with propofol using the Marsh model*

This is illustrated in Figure 10, p. 38, which shows the simulated infusion profiles, and predicted blood concentrations (in a 70 kg patient) if the Marsh model is used for administering an effect-site targeted infusion, but with two different keo values. For both curves the target concentration is set at 4 μg/ml at time zero, and then reduced to 2 μg/ml at 10 minutes. As can be seen from the graphs the blood concentrations required to achieve these target effect-site concentrations are highly sensitive to the choice of k_{eo} or $t_{1/2} k_{eo}$.

At present two different values are commonly used with the Marsh model for propofol. The first is a $t_{1/2} k_{eo}$ of 2.6 min, equivalent to a k_{eo} of 0.26 min^{-1} (as implemented in the Diprifusor, and used for displaying estimated effect-site concentrations). This value was based on a study by Billard and colleagues[123] who found a k_{eo} of 0.2 min^{-1}. The second is a t1/2 k_{eo} of 34 sec, equivalent to a k_{eo} of 1.2 min^{-1}, based on a time to peak effect of 1.6 min.[124] This "faster" k_{eo} value has been recommended for use in combination with the Marsh model forming the "Modified Marsh model",[124] as implemented by two new "open-TCI systems" the "Base Primea" (Fresenius, Brezins, France) and the "Asena PK" (Alaris Medical Systems, Basingstoke, UK).

When a "slow" k_{eo} is used, an increase in target effect-site concentration will require higher blood drug concentrations to generate a bigger gradient to drive

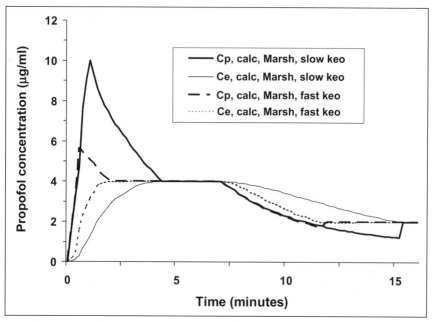

Figure 10: Effect-site targeted TCI for propofol using the Marsh model, showing the effect of the choice of k_{eo}. The thick lines illustrate the required target blood concentrations for k_{eo} values of 0.26 ("slow") and 1.2 min^{-1} ("fast") respectively

the drug into the effect-site. It can be seen from Figure 10 that when the "slow" k_{eo} (0.26 min^{-1}) is used the peak blood propofol concentration required to quickly produce an effect-site concentration of 4 µg/ml is just over 9 µg/ml, whereas if the "fast" k_{eo} (1.2 min^{-1}, equivalent to a t1/2 k_{eo} of 34 sec), the peak blood concentration required is less than 6 µg/ml and the total dose administered by 10 min is 3 ml less. Conversely, when the target concentration is reduced, the "slow" k_{eo} will require the blood concentrations to fall further to minimise the time taken for the effect-site concentration to reach the new target.

In fit young patients "slow" k_{eo} values are less likely to cause problems, whereas in the elderly the large overshoots may result in adverse effects such as cardiovascular instability. Thus if effect-site targeting is used in elderly patients it is safer to use a faster k_{eo}.

7.1.2. Effect-site targeting with propofol using the Schnider model

The Schnider model is usually used in effect-site targeted infusions of propofol. As mentioned before, it is a more complex model than the Marsh model, as it incorporates age, height, weight, and lean body mass (which is calculated from an equation using height, weight and gender as variables – see earlier section called "Which figure for patient weight should be used for TCI and TIVA" for a more detailed discussion). During the study by Schnider and colleagues it was determined that the time to peak effect (TTPE) for propofol in their study was 1.6 min. This figure is used to calculate an individualised k_{eo} value for each patient. This is illustrated in figure 11 which shows the time course of blood and effect-site concentrations predicted by the Schnider model following a 2 mg/kg propofol bolus administered to two different male patients who both weigh 70 kg. For an 18 year old patient who is 160 cm tall the TTPE method (using a TTPE of 1.6 min) will result in a k_{eo} of 0.357, whereas for an 80 year old man who is 180 cm tall the k_{eo} will be 0.525.

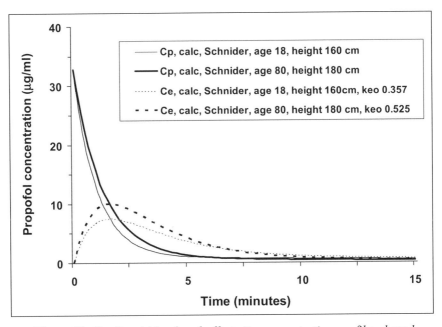

Figure 11: Predicted blood and effect-site concentration profiles, based on the Schnider model and a TTPE of 1.6 min, for two different patients who both weigh 70 kg and who have each received a 2 mg/kg intravenous bolus dose of propofol

A TTPE of 1.6 min implies a much quicker time to maximum effect-site concentrations and clinical effects after a bolus than the value implicit in the Marsh model (the k_{eo} value of 0.26 min^{-1} used by the Marsh model equates to a TTPE of 4.57 min). Thus when the Schnider model is used for effect-site targeting, relatively less "overshoot" and "undershoot" of blood concentrations around the target effect-site concentration is required. For this reason, and also because of the pharmacokinetic parameters used in the Schnider model, effect-site targeting using the Schnider model results in lower doses of propofol than when the Marsh model is used for blood concentration targeting, and in the elderly or compromised patient, this may result in better cardiovascular stability (see later section "Differences between Marsh and Schnider models").

7.2. *Effect-site targeted opioid infusions*

It is theoretically possible to administer effect-site targeted TCI infusions of opioids for which k_{eo} values have been calculated or for which the TTPE is known; and when step-wise changes in effect-site opioid concentrations are required or desirable, effect-site targeting may be useful. There are a few problems with effect-site targeting of opioids. The first is that there have been few combined pharmacokinetic-dynamic studies. For most of the opioids, the k_{eo} values that have been published have been determined from pure pharmacodynamic studies in which the measure of clinical effect was one or more of the parameters derived from the spontaneous EEG (such as SEF and MF). These parameters have not been conclusively shown to correlate with clinical indicators of analgesia.

For remifentanil, Minto and colleagues did perform a formal combined pharmacokinetic and dynamic study. The k_{eo} that they derived is adjusted for age as follows: $k_{eo} = 0.595 - 0.007 \times (age - 40)$.[53] For alfentanil a k_{eo} value of 0.77 min^{-1} is sometimes used to calculate effect-site concentrations. This value, also used by Maitre and colleagues in their study of the pharmacokinetics of alfentanil,[63] was determined from a study performed by Scott et al.[125] For sufentanil, the k_{eo} value of 0.119 min^{-1} calculated by Scott and colleagues[126] is sometimes used with the Gepts model to calculate effect-site concentrations.

When a k_{eo} is used during blood concentration targeted infusions to simply estimate the effect-site concentration, errors are less clinically significant. As mentioned earlier, during effect-site targeted infusions the choice of k_{eo} is more critical, because it will significantly affect the rate of infusion of drug after a change in target concentration. Given that TTPE values for sufentanil and alfentanil have been published (5.4 and 1.4 min respectively),[127] it is probably better to use a TTPE method to calculate individualised k_{eo} values when effect-site targeted infusions of sufentanil and alfentanil are administered.

So, is effect-site targeting really necessary for the opiates? In the case of remifentanil, the case for effect-site targeting is less compelling, because simulations show that when using a blood targeted infusion, equilibration between blood and effect-site concentrations is virtually complete within 5 mins. With blood concentration targeting, rapid rises in effect-site concentration can be achieved by brief periods of overshoot. When effect-site targeting is used, the overshoot is of course calculated and controlled automatically. Because the blood concentration of remifentanil falls so rapidly after an infusion stops, an effect-site targeted remifentanil infusion system is able to choose very high target blood concentrations, and in doing so to achieve almost step-wise increases in estimated effect-site concentrations. Although the overshoot will only be temporary it is worth bearing in mind, or placing a limit of the degree of overshoot. If the Minto model is used for effect-site targeting, and the overshoot is not limited, an initial effect-site target of 6 ng/ml will require a peak blood concentration of 17 ng/ml, a level that may be associated with adverse effects such as chest wall rigidity and bradycardias in compromised patients.

The argument is somewhat stronger for opioids that do not equilibrate as rapidly with the effect-site, such as sufentanil. With these drugs, effect-site targeting will hasten the onset of clinical effect. At present there is little scientific evidence that effect-site targeting is superior to blood targeting for target-controlled opioid infusions. It is difficult to find compelling reasons for using effect-site targeted (or even blood concentration targeted) infusions of opioids such as morphine and fentanyl that accumulate because of slow metabolism and/or large volumes of distribution.

III. Pharmacodynamics

1. General

Pharmacodynamics describes the relationship between blood concentration of a drug and clinical effect; and so is often said to describe "what the drug does to the body." In the following section the range of therapeutic concentrations for various drugs will be outlined. Because of the wide variability in individual patient pharmacokinetics and pharmacodynamics, and pharmacodynamic and pharmacokinetic interactions between co-administered drugs (discussed further below) no single regimen, concentration or drug combination applies to all patients. A dose that is excessive for one patient may be inadequate for the next. As with inhalational anaesthesia clinical judgement is always required, and the doses of drugs used should be titrated according to the clinical response of the patient.

As alluded to earlier, the significance of the effect-site compartment has only been fully appreciated in recent years. Thus many earlier studies that reported therapeutic concentration ranges referred only to blood concentrations, whereas the estimated effect-site concentration is probably of greater significance.

2. Overview of the pharmacodynamics of commonly used anaesthetic agents

2.1. Propofol

2.1.1. Sedation

Propofol at low doses is associated with a pleasant feeling (bordering on euphoria), anxiolysis and sedation. The blood and effect-site concentrations required to achieve these effects vary markedly among patients.

Studies using patient-maintained sedation (PMS) systems provide the most objective evidence of the likely dose requirements for sedation, because they allow the patient to control the dose (target concentration of a TCI system). When a patient using one of these systems presses the activating button after a lockout period, the system increases the target concentration by a pre-defined amount, and thus administers a target-controlled infusion to maintain the concentration at that level. In a study performed by Irwin, 39 patients used a PMS system, to self-administer propofol for sedation during orthopaedic surgery under local or regional anaesthesia.[128] They self-administered a median blood propofol concentration of 0.8-0.9 µg/ml. The mean infusion rate was 2.4 (range 0.18-7.9) mg/kg/hr. No patient lost consciousness.

In another study the same system was used to provide 45 min of "instant pre-medication" for 20 patients awaiting day case surgery.[129] Median target blood propofol concentrations at 15, 30 and 45 min varied between 1.0 and 1.3 µg/ml, and the mean propofol infusion rate was 3 mg/kg/hr. There were significant reductions in anxiety scores, and no episodes of cardiovascular instability or excessive sedation (all continued to respond to voice).

Two studies of the safety of the system have been performed in healthy (unstimulated) volunteers. In both studies the volunteers were encouraged to operate the system repetitively in an attempt to anaesthetise themselves.[130,131] At maximal sedation, when the volunteers were too sedated to press the button of the activating handset, the median target propofol concentration in the first study (10 volunteers) was 2.0 (range 1.4 to 3) µg/ml, and the mean propofol infusion rate was 5.3 mg/kg/hr. Two volunteers became oversedated (one did not respond to painful stimuli), but in both cases the target blood concentration was only 1.4 µg/ml.[130] In the second study (16 volunteers), using a different starting concentration and lockout period, the median blood propofol concentration at maximal sedation was 1.7 (range 1-2.5) µg/ml. All volunteers remained conscious throughout, but one suffered a brief episode of apnoea at an estimate blood concentration of 1.0 µg/ml.[131]

In a recent study TCI propofol was used for sedation in 122 adult patients on 6 intensive care units (along with morphine, fentanyl or alfentanil for analgesia).[132] The median target propofol concentration used was 1.34 µg/ml in post-cardiac surgery patients, 0.98 µg/ml in brain injured adults and 0.42 µg/ml in general intensive care patients. The mean average propofol infusion rate was 1.8 mg/kg/hr (range 0.2-4.8 mg/kg/hr).

2.1.2. Induction of anaesthesia

In unpremedicated patients in whom no other anaesthetic agents are administered, the mean blood propofol concentration required for loss of consciousness is of the order of 5-6 µg/ml.[36,40] However, in elderly or unwell patients the starting blood propofol concentration should be less than this. In patients who have received a sedative premedication or those in whom propofol is supplemented by nitrous oxide or an opioid, blood concentrations in the range 4-5 µg/ml are required.[29,36,40] Measured blood concentrations in the range 1.0 to 2.19 µg/ml have been recorded in volunteers when waking from anaesthesia.[133]

More recently, Struys et al, using the Schnider model, found that the $Ce_{50,\,LOC}$ (effect-site propofol concentration required for loss of eyelash reflex in 50% of patients) was 2.9 µg/ml if only propofol was used, 1.8 µg/ml in the presence of remifentanil 2 ng/ml and 1.7 µg/ml in the presence of remifentanil 4 ng/ml.[134]

2.1.3. Maintenance of anaesthesia

Published propofol concentrations required to prevent a response to a noxious stimulus gives some indication of the concentrations required for maintenance of anaesthesia during surgical procedures. Studies by Stuart and Davidson found that the plasma propofol concentration required to prevent purposeful movement in response to surgical incision in 50% of patients (C_{p50}) is of the order of 6-7 µg/ml in un-premedicated patients not receiving nitrous oxide, and 4-5 µg/ml in un-premedicated patients receiving 67% nitrous oxide.[101,135] Struys and colleagues reported that the C_{e50} for preventing a response to noxious stimuli was 4.1 µg/ml when only propofol was used, 1.8 µg/ml when remifentanil 2 ng/ml was administered and 1.7 µg/ml when remifentanil 4 ng/ml was administered.[134]

These concentrations are all well above those reported for inhibition of learning and memory functions. Using a Trivial Pursuit learning task Leslie and colleagues found that a measured blood propofol concentration of 0.66 µg/ml inhibited learning in 50% of volunteers.[136]

2.2. Remifentanil

Most of the published information refers to the use of remifentanil in association with TCI propofol or an inhalational agent for induction and maintenance of anaesthesia in ventilated adult patients. The remifentanil target concentrations used reflect the synergistic pharmacodynamic interaction between remifentanil and hypnotic agents.[137] In association with these agents, adequate analgesia for surgery has generally been achieved with target blood remifentanil concentrations in the range of 3 to 8 ng/ml with titration of the target setting against the response of the patient. For particularly stimulating procedures target concentrations up to 15 ng/ml have been used safely.

Simulations show that with frequently used remifentanil infusion rates of 0.25 to 0.5 µg/kg/min in a 70 kg, 170 cm, 40 year old patient, the calculated remifentanil blood concentration approaches steady state after 25 min at concentrations of 6.3 to 12.6 ng/ml.

2.3. Sufentanil

Sufentanil has been used as a mono-anaesthetic agent during cardiac surgery. Under these circumstances Bailey found very high measured plasma levels of sufentanil (> 20 ng/ml).[138] In more recent studies using TCI sufentanil with the Gepts model in combination of propofol, isoflurane and midazolam, the target blood concentrations used were between 1 and 10 ng/ml during cardiac surgery[103,105] and between 0.1 and 1 ng/ml during general surgery.[104,106] In some countries, recommended concentrations are included in the drug label. In France the drug label recommends target concentrations between 0.4 and 2 ng/ml for cardiac surgery, and between 0.15 and 0.6 ng/ml for non-cardiac surgery. In the latest version of Miller's Anesthesia, therapeutic concentrations of sufentanil are described as follows: predominant or sole agent 5-10 ng/ml; major surgery 1-3 ng/ml; minor surgery 0.3-0.6 ng/ml; spontaneous ventilation < 0.4 ng/ml.[139]

2.4. Alfentanil

Numerous publications have described ranges of "therapeutic concentrations" for alfentanil. Several of the older publications by Ausems reported the alfentanil concentrations required to prevent responses to noxious stimuli when it was used with nitrous oxide and no other hypnotic. These studies reported Cp50 values for intubation and skin incision of 475 and 279 ng/ml respectively.[140-142] These high values probably reflect the low hypnotic potency of nitrous oxide.

Vuyk has studied the pharmacodynamics of alfentanil as a supplement to either propofol or N_2O during lower abdominal surgery in female patients.[143] In this study, fixed concentrations of either propofol (3 µg/ml) or nitrous oxide (66%) were administered, while the target concentration of TCI alfentanil was adjusted according to patient responses. The Cp50 values for alfentanil in combination with propofol were 92 ng/ml for intubation, 55 ng/ml for skin incision, 84 ng/ml for peritoneal incision, and 66 ng/ml for the intra-abdominal part of surgery. The corresponding values during nitrous oxide anaesthesia were significantly higher: 429 ng/ml for intubation, 101 ng/ml for skin incision, and 206 ng/ml for the intra-abdominal part of surgery.

3. Pharmacodynamic interactions

A pharmacodynamic interaction is said to occur when the use of a combination of agents results in a change in the clinical effect from that which would have occurred if either agent had been used on its own. Little is known about the mechanism of pharmacodynamic interactions. Additive or supra-additive pharmacodynamic interactions between most classes of anaesthetic agents have been found. Opioids, benzodiazepines, clonidine and even esmolol have all been shown to reduce the dose requirements of intravenous and inhalational hypnotic agents.[144-155] **Pharmacodynamic** interactions tend to be far more significant, and potent, than **pharmacokinetic** interactions. The most widely studied interactions are those between opioids and propofol.

In the previous section the study by Vuyk et al of the influence of propofol on the alfentanil dose required to prevent responses to intraoperative noxious stimuli was discussed. The same authors later performed another study of the pharmacodynamic interaction between propofol and alfentanil, during which the patients received one of four fixed concentrations of alfentanil, while propofol concentrations were adjusted.[156] This study enabled the authors to determine measured blood propofol concentrations associated with different end points, at different alfentanil concentrations. These endpoints included loss and return of consciousness, and 10% reductions in blood pressure and heart rates. A similar, more recent study has investigated the pharmacodynamic interaction between propofol and remifentanil (again examining responses to noxious stimuli, and concentrations associated with loss and return of consciousness).[137]

Struys and colleagues found a similar degree of synergism for propofol and remifentanil with regard to loss of response to noxious stimuli during induction of anaesthesia.[134] They also examined the interaction with regard to loss of eyelash reflex, and loss of response to verbal command. As expected, given the potent analgesic effects of remifentanil, the synergism between remifentanil and propofol was most profound for response to painful stimuli – a blood remifentanil concentration of 4 ng/ml reduced the Cp50 for loss of response to verbal command from 2.9 to 2.2 µg/ml; whereas it reduced the Cp50 for loss of response to noxious stimulus from 4.1 to 1.3 µg/ml. What was more interesting and unexpected is that in the presence of a modest dose of remifentanil, the propofol Cp50 for response to pain was lower than that required for both response to verbal command and for loss of eyelash reflex.

Combinations of agents that result in supra-additive clinical effects offer significant benefits for patients. They enable the anaesthetist to achieve clinically equivalent levels of anaesthesia with lower total doses of drugs. In general the hypnotic agents (inhalational and intravenous) tend to have more profound effects on cardiovascular parameters (such as blood pressure, systemic resistance and cardiac output) than the opioids. Thus when a combination of a hypnotic and an opioid is used, the dose of hypnotic can be reduced to enhance cardiovascular stability, which is especially beneficial in patients with limited cardiac reserves.

Different opioids have very different pharmacokinetic profiles, and so when they are used in combination with a hypnotic agent, they will affect the rate at which consciousness is regained when the anaesthetic administration ceases. The rate at which a patient will regain consciousness thus depends on the choice of agents, the respective doses, the sensitivity of the patient to the effects of the agents and in the case of agents whose elimination is context-sensitive, the duration of infusions of the agents used. If two agents are used in combination, then the fastest possible recovery can be achieved if a higher dose of the agent with the quickest "offset" is used in combination with a lower dose of the "slower" agent.

Vuyk et al have used computer simulations to extrapolate the data from his propofol/alfentanil interaction study[156] to other opioids, so that they were able to publish optimal combinations of propofol with other opioids that they estimated would not only prevent responses to noxious stimuli in 50% and 95% of patients, but would also result in the fastest recovery from anaesthesia.[157]

So far this section on interactions has concentrated on the potentiation of the effects of hypnotic agents on conscious levels. The Vuyk group has also studied the pharmacodynamic interactions of propofol and remifentanil with regard to control of breathing.[158] They found that even at low concentrations of propofol and remifentanil (levels at which many patients will not have lost consciousness) the respiratory drive, as assessed by CO_2 sensitivity and minute ventilation, was almost completely eliminated.

Bouillon et al have recently studied the pharmacodynamic interaction between propofol and remifentanil, with the endpoints being response to shaking, shouting and laryngoscopy.[159] Their findings confirm the dramatic synergism between the two agents. While remifentanil alone did not ablate the responses to laryngoscopy, and even to shaking and shouting, propofol in higher doses was able to do so. Modest concentrations of remifentanil cause a large reduction in the target propofol concentrations required to ablate the responses.

IV. Practical aspects

1. Manual infusion regimens

In this section some standardised manual infusion regimens will be described to assist those who do not have access to TCI technology, or who prefer, for whatever reason, to use manually controlled infusions. With these regimens it is possible to achieve steady state blood concentrations quite quickly, but unfortunately the concentrations achieved will not be suitable for all patients. A blood or effect-site concentration that is too high for one patient may be too low for another, so that the regimens cannot be blindly followed, but should rather be used as a starting point from which infusion rates are adjusted according to the needs of the individual patient. Titrating to effect can be more precisely and rapidly performed with TCI systems, whereas the best the anaesthetist can do when titrating a manually controlled infusion is to have an educated guess at the sizes of boluses or infusion rate changes that need to be made to sufficiently increase or decrease the blood and effect-site concentration of an anaesthetic drug.

1.1. Propofol

Before the advent of target-controlled infusion systems several manual infusion schemes aiming to achieve steady state propofol concentrations, were proposed. One of the most commonly used schemes was that proposed by Roberts and colleagues,[160] which gives a fairly close approximation to a steady state concentration of 3 µg/ml. It is worth remembering that this regimen is insufficient for use without analgesic or other agents during surgery. Close inspection of the original description reveals that Roberts and colleges administered 3 µg/kg of fentanyl before starting the propofol infusion, and then mechanically ventilated the lungs of their patients with 67% N_2O.

This infusion scheme involves an initial bolus of 1 mg/kg at induction followed by 10 mg/kg/hr for 10minutes, then 8 mg/kg/hr for 10 minutes and finally 6 mg/kg/hr. Figure 12, p. 50, shows the resulting blood concentrations estimated using the Marsh model.[42] The estimated blood concentration reaches a nadir of 2.7 µg/ml after half an hour. Thereafter it increases only slowly, eventually reaching a steady state concentration of 3.6 µg/ml after about 24 hours. If the Schnider model[45] is used to estimate the blood concentrations, the estimated blood concentrations soon after the bolus are significantly higher (see below and Figure 13, p. 51), whereas later the differences between the estimations of the Marsh and Schnider models is much smaller.

For either model complete equilibration between compartments is estimated to have occurred by 24 hours. For the Schnider model the estimated blood concentration at equilibrium is 4.1 µg/ml.

Because the kinetics of propofol are generally linear, a proportional change to the size of the initial bolus and subsequent infusion rates will result in a proportional change (of similar magnitude) in blood concentration achieved. Thus an anaesthetist wishing to adjust the Robert infusion regime to achieve a different target concentration should make a proportional adjustment to the bolus dose and infusion rates. As mentioned earlier, while this sort of regimen can easily be used to achieve (close to) steady state blood concentrations, it is not easy to accurately achieve different magnitudes of proportional change to the target concentration over time. Rapid changes in blood concentration can only be achieved by boluses. A simple rule of thumb is that, according to the Marsh model, 1 mg/kg bolus given to a healthy adult patient will increase the blood propofol concentration by 4 µg/ml. Thus, if the Roberts regime has been followed for more than 20 minutes, and the anaesthetist wishes to increase the blood concentration from ~3 g/ml to ~4 µg/ml, then a bolus of 0.25 mg/kg followed by an infusion at 7.5 mg/kg/hr is required.

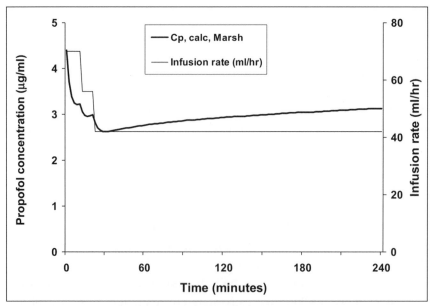

Figure 12: The "Roberts" manual propofol infusion regimen, showing the estimated blood concentrations as predicted by the Marsh model. After 4 hours the estimated concentration is just over 3 µg/ml. Complete equilibration and steady state are only reached after 24 hours

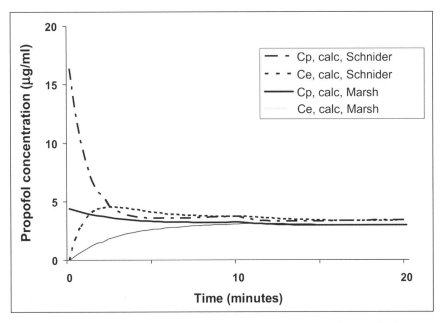

Figure 13: Blood and effect-site propofol concentrations during the first 30 min of use of the Roberts infusion regimen, as estimated by the Marsh and Schnider models for a 70 kg male, height 170 cm

1.2. Remifentanil

Prior to the recent introduction of open TCI systems, few anaesthetists had access to infusion systems programmed to deliver TCI remifentanil. Thus most anaesthetists using remifentanil will have developed their own manual infusion "recipe" for using it.

When remifentanil was first released the manufacturer (GlaxoWellcome, UK) issued very broad dosing guidelines for induction bolus sizes, and for maintenance infusion rates. Anaesthetists who used remifentanil at the upper limits of the bolus and infusion rate recommendations soon found that those doses were commonly associated with adverse effects such as bradycardias and chest wall rigidity.

For induction of anaesthesia, a commonly used regimen is to give an infusion of 0.5 µg/kg/min for 3 min, followed by an infusion of 0.25 µg/kg/min. With this regimen steady state blood concentrations result after about 20 min (approximately 6 ng/ml in younger patients, and 9 ng/ml in elderly patients – see Figure 6, p. 29). As can be seen inferred from Figure 6, it takes a few minutes before therapeutic effect-site concentrations will be achieved with this regimen. If a more rapid onset of action is desired then a bolus dose can be given, but to avoid adverse events, it should always be given slowly. One approach is to administer the bolus "on top of" the initial infusion rate over 1 minute. Using the regimens described above, an anaesthetist wishing to administer a careful bolus may set the pump to deliver an infusion at 1 µg/kg/min for 1 minute, then reduce the rate to 0.5 µg/kg/min for a further 2 min before making further reductions in infusion rate. This regimen will result in an almost step-wise increase in blood concentration to ~6 ng/ml. Fit, young patients will usually tolerate this regimen very well. The bolus dose should be halved in elderly patients, and omitted in those who are very frail or unwell. In fit young patients maintenance infusion rates of between 0.12 and 0.5 µg/kg/min usually suffice (rates higher than that are rarely needed). Once again these rates should be reduced in the elderly (typically infusion rates between 0.08 and 0.25 µg/kg/min are sufficient).

1.3. Sufentanil

Glass et al have recommended manual infusion schemes for sufentanil.[139] For sedation or analgesia, a loading dose of between 0.1 and 0.5 µg/kg, followed by an infusion of 0.005-0.01 µg/kg/min is recommended and should generate a blood concentration of approximately 0.2 ng/ml. For general anaesthesia Glass recommend a loading dose of 1-5 µg/kg followed by an infusion at 0.01-0.05 µg/kg/min. After an initial overshoot this regimen should generate blood concentrations between 0.6 and 3 ng/ml. However, clinical experience shows that concentrations between 0.1 and 0.4 ng/ml are sufficient for most operations, and that higher concentrations are only required during cardiac surgery.

1.4. Ketamine

When ketamine is the sole agent used for induction of anaesthesia, bolus doses of between 1 and 2 mg/kg are required. A bolus dose of 2 mg/kg will typically produce 10-15 minutes of anaesthesia. For maintenance, infusion rates of 1-2 mg/kg/hr are needed. A bolus dose of 2 mg/kg followed by an infusion at 2 mg/kg/hr will result in concentrations estimated to be ~700-800 ng/ml depending on the model used to predict the concentrations (Clements: 700 ng/ml; Domino ~800 ng/ml).

When ketamine is being used as an adjunct to another hypnotic agent, lower doses are required. Typical doses recommended for an anti-hyperalgesic effect are an infusion at 0.5 mg/kg/hr. If no bolus is given, blood concentrations will increase for several hours. After 60 minutes, several hours before steady state is reached, the Domino model will estimate blood concentrations of ~170 ng/ml, whereas the Clements model will estimate concentrations of ~140 ng/ml.

2. Induction and maintenance of anaesthesia with TCI propofol

2.1. Blood-targeted TCI

The first generation of commercially available ('Diprifusor' – containing) propofol TCI pumps only offered blood targeted TCI, and thus this is the TCI mode that most anaesthetists will be familiar with.

If there is likely to be a time delay between venous cannulation and induction of anaesthesia (e.g while final preparations and checks are made) then it is worth starting the infusion at a low target concentration (1-1.5 µg/ml in a fit young patient) as soon as possible. Not only does this provide further anxiolysis at an otherwise stressful time, it also gives the anaesthetist a chance to judge the individual patient's sensitivity to the effects of propofol. This 'instant' pre-medication with propofol may well also reduce the dose required for loss of consciousness.

When the anaesthetist wishes to induce anaesthesia, it is usually best to choose an initial *blood* target concentration that is above the anticipated *effect-site* concentration required for loss of consciousness, to cause the effect-site concentration to rise more quickly (analogous to use of "overpressure" with inhalational anaesthetic agents). If anaesthesia is not lost within a minute or two, incremental increases in target blood concentration may be required. Once consciousness has been lost and the airway secured, the target blood concentration should be reduced to a value close to the effect-site concentration at that time.

Typical blood propofol concentrations required for loss of consciousness in fit young patients are of the order of 6-8 µg/ml. Patients who are very anxious, have not received a sedative premedication and/or are not also having an opioid bolus for induction, may require even higher target concentrations for loss of consciousness. In these patients it is probably acceptable to start at target concentrations of 6 µg/ml, and then adjust the target upwards every 30 sec as required. In middle-aged patients and elderly patients it is better to start induction with target concentrations of ~4 µg/ml. Naturally even greater caution should be exercised if the patient is unwell or is likely to suffer cardiovascular instability, in which cases it is advisable to start at much lower concentrations, such as 1.5 µg/ml, and wait a minute of two before slowly increasing the target concentration in 0.5 µg/ml steps (see advice below).

When consciousness is lost, and again during manipulation of the airway (tracheal intubation or laryngeal mask insertion) it is advisable to take note of the estimated effect-site propofol concentration to give further "calibration points" for the patient's sensitivity to propofol. For example if the blood pressure and heart rate do not change during tracheal intubation then it is safe to assume that the effect-site concentration at that time was adequate for a noxious stimulus. Once stable anaesthesia is achieved, the anaesthetist may need to consider reducing the target blood concentration towards the current estimated effect-site concentration.

During the case the patient should be observed closely. The target concentrations used should be adjusted according to the clinical responses of the patient, and will also be influenced by the co-administration of other agents that influence depth of anaesthesia such as ketamine, opioids, nitrous oxide and benzodiazepines. Towards the end of the case, as the intensity of the surgical stimulus reduces, the target concentrations can be gradually reduced to promote a more rapid recovery from anaesthesia. Generally the infusion can be stopped (by changing the target concentration to zero) once the final sutures or dressings are applied.

2.2. Effect-site targeted TCI

When effect-site targeting is used there is of course no need for use of "overpressure" to increase the effect-site concentrations more rapidly during induction, because the infusion pump is doing this automatically. If, as mentioned before, there is likely to be a delay between insertion of a venous cannula and induction of anaesthesia, it is worth starting at a low target concentration (approximately 0.5 µg/ml) to provide some anxiolysis and to enable an assessment of the sensitivity of the patient to propofol. After that, when the anaesthetist wishes to induce anaesthesia, the target can be set at a level that he estimates will be sufficient for loss of consciousness. Once the target effect-site concentration is reached, the clinical effect should be assessed, and the target increased or decreased as required. Naturally, if the patient is elderly or unwell, or the anaesthetist wishes to exercise caution for whatever reason, then it is wise to increase the target concentration in smaller steps during induction of anaesthesia.

After induction, the target concentration should be increased or decreased, as appropriate for the level of surgical and other stimuli. If, for example, there is a long delay after induction of anaesthesia, while the surgeons prepare themselves and the patient then it may be appropriate to reduce the target concentration temporarily. In general it may be wise, during a painful surgical procedure, to select an effect-site concentration target at least as high as that present during laryngoscopy (and even higher if there was a haemodynamic response during laryngoscopy).

2.3. Differences between Marsh and Schnider models

Most anaesthetists interested in intravenous anaesthesia will be aware of the pharmacokinetic models for propofol published by Marsh[42] and Schnider.[45] Many will have used one or other model, when administering propofol TCI. Use of a TCI system does not, however, imply or require an intimate knowledge of the model used by the system. Anaesthetists who are accustomed to using one model to control a propofol TCI should exercise caution before using another model, and be certain that the differences between the models are understood. Computer simulations can be used to understand the differences in estimated concentrations achieved when equivalent doses are administered, and more importantly the differences in dose administered when the different models are used to control a TCI, before proceeding with caution, preferably in a fit, healthy patient who does not require muscle relaxation.

One major difference between the Marsh and Schnider models is the size of the central compartment. For a patient who weighs 70 kg, the Marsh model will use a Vc value of 15.9 L whereas the corresponding value for the Schnider model is 4.27 L. As mentioned earlier the Schnider model uses this figure for all patients. Because of this difference, the estimated concentrations following boluses or rapid infusions vary greatly. Figure 13 illustrates the blood and effect-site concentrations estimated by the two models for the first 30 min when the "Roberts" manual regimen[138] for propofol is used (1 mg/kg bolus, followed by an infusion at 10 mg/kg/hr for 10 min, then at 8 mg/kg/hr for a further 10 min, and finally at 6 mg/kg/hr – also see Figure 13). There are striking differences in the estimated blood and effect-site concentrations for the first 10 min after the bolus. One minute after the bolus the Marsh model will result in estimated blood and effect-site concentrations of 4.0 and 0.9 µg/ml respectively, whereas the corresponding values for the Schnider model will be 8.2 and 3.6 µg/ml respectively. After 10 min the differences become less significant. At 30 min, the Marsh parameters will result in an estimated blood and effect-site concentration of 2.7 g/ml, whereas the corresponding values with the Schnider model are 3.0 µg/ml.

When propofol administration is stopped, large differences in the estimated concentrations are again found (Figure 14), with the Schnider model estimating a much more rapid fall in concentrations than the Marsh model. This is mostly because the Schnider model has a smaller Vc, a larger k10 (i.e. "faster" metabolic clearance) and a larger keo (i.e. "faster" equilibration between central and effect-site compartments).

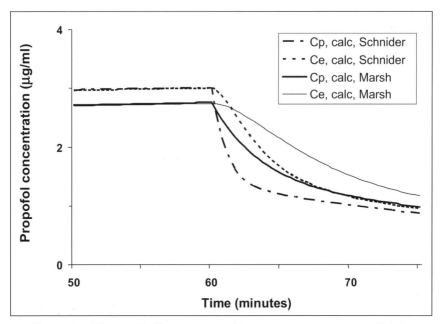

Figure 14: Blood and effect-site propofol concentrations estimated by the Marsh and Schnider models when the Roberts infusion regimen is stopped after 60 min in a 70 kg adult male, height 170 cm

When propofol is administered by TCI, and the Schnider model is used, the nett effect of these differences is that less propofol is administered. Figure 15, p. 57, illustrates the cumulative volume of 1% propofol infused when the Marsh and Schnider models are used for a TCI propofol infusion at a target concentration fixed at 4 µg/ml, and shows that even when the Schnider model is used in *effect-site* targeted mode, it will result in a lower cumulative propofol dose than the Marsh model in *blood* targeted mode. The biggest difference in infusion rates occurs during the first few minutes after an increase in target concentration. With the passage of time the significance of the difference in infusion rates diminishes.

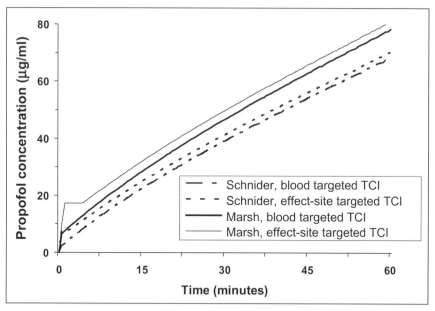

Figure 15: Comparison of the cumulative dose of propofol 1% infused when a TCI system uses the Marsh and Schnider models at a target blood concentration of 4 µg/ml

During induction of anaesthesia with the Schnider model, anaesthetists more familiar with the Marsh model will find that for a given target concentration, the onset of clinical effects will occur more slowly than if the Marsh model were used. If a more rapid induction of anaesthesia is required (i.e. a larger initial bolus) then it will be necessary to use a higher initial target concentration. Practically speaking, when an anaesthetist who is more familiar with the Marsh model starts using the Schnider model, he/she should remember to always use the Schnider model in effect-site targeting mode, and should use somewhat higher initial target concentrations than he would have with the Marsh model.

Likewise, an anaesthetist more familiar with the Schnider model will find that when the Marsh model is used, the larger initial bolus results in more rapid clinical effects (at a given target concentration) and may be associated with more severe adverse effects. This is particularly true for elderly patients, for whom the Schnider model is more "gentle" as it makes allowances for the reduced rate of distribution clearance between the Vc and V2 found in elderly patients.

3. Advice for the complete TIVA novice

Anaesthetists wishing to use intravenous maintenance of anaesthesia for the first time should choose their first cases carefully, and not jump directly in the "deep end." As with all clinical skills, there are many different ways of achieving the same goal, albeit during learning or during clinical practise. The advice that follows should be followed in a general sense, bearing in mind that all patients are different, doses should always be titrated to clinical effect, and of course there are remarkable differences in practise between different hospitals and different countries. Please do not apply the examples given here as fixed recipes!

The safest way to acquire some basic clinical skills in intravenous anaesthesia is to start by using propofol infusions (either manually controlled, or using TCI system) for procedural sedation or for sedation during surgical procedures performed under local or regional anaesthesia. Start a TCI propofol system at an initial target of 0.5 µg/ml (using either the Marsh model in blood targeted mode, or the Schnider model in effect-site targeted mode), then wait and observe the clinical effect for a few minutes. After that adjust the target concentration in small steps (0.1-0.2 µg/ml increments or decrements), observing the patient closely between steps. Remember that the dose or target concentration required will change if other drugs are used, and as the intensity of any noxious stimulus changes. When manual regimens are used for propofol sedation, anaesthetists will typically administer small boluses of ~10-20 mg and use an infusion rate of the order of 3 mg/kg/hr.

When progressing on to use TIVA for the first time for general anaesthesia we would recommend starting with a minor surgical case in a fit patient aged 20-40, in whom spontaneous ventilation via a laryngeal mask airway (LMA) is feasible, and for which local or regional anaesthesia is possible. There are many such cases; examples include operations for ingrown toenails, tendon or nerve repairs and varicose veins.

If a propofol TCI system is available then it is probably best to use it, and either use the Marsh model in blood targeted mode, or the Schnider model in effect-site targeted mode. Second best is an infusion pump that will allow the user to enter the infusion rate in mg/kg/hr, to enable the user to administer a variant of the Roberts regimen. If a monitor of anaesthetic depth is available then it should be used for further reassurance, and the electrodes applied for induction of anaesthesia. Before starting the propofol infusion, inject 2-3 ml of 1% lidocaine to attenuate any pain at the start of the propofol infusion. Two minutes before starting the propofol administer a modest intravenous dose of fentanyl or alfentanil (eg. 1 µg/kg fentanyl, or 10 µg/kg alfentanil). If using a TCI system, start the infusion at a target concentration of 4 µg/ml. Once this concentration has been achieved, assess the conscious state of the patient continuously, and increase the target concentration in steps of 0.5 µg/ml until the patient no longer responds to voice and the eyelash reflex is lost. Observe the effect-site concentration at loss of consciousness. Once the patient's jaw is sufficiently relaxed, attempt LMA insertion. If the jaw is not relaxed, or the patient resists LMA insertion, wait a little longer, and increase the target concentration if necessary.

Once the LMA has been inserted, again observe the effect-site propofol concentration – at this stage it is probably still significantly lower than the estimated blood concentration. Reduce the target blood concentration to the same, or a slightly higher level than the effect-site concentration. Assist ventilation manually until spontaneous ventilation returns, using 30-40% O_2 in air; or if you usually use N_2O (and work in an unfortunate place where it is still is allowed) then use a mixture of 60-70% N_2O in 30-40% O_2. If feasible perform a nerve or field local anaesthetic block.

"Invite" the surgeon to start the operation once you are confident the patient is adequately anaesthetised, cardiovascular parameters are stable, and the exhaled N_2O concentration is at least 40% (if used). If the patient becomes tachypnoeic, or tachycardic, increase the target propofol concentration, and consider administering another modest dose of fentanyl or alfentanil. If the blood pressure is low, and the patient remains apnoeic for longer than expected, it may be necessary to reduce the target propofol concentration.

When the surgeon is starting to close the wound, reduce the target propofol concentration by ~25%; once the last suture is in place, switch off the infusion and the nitrous oxide, and observe the rapid and clear-headed recovery of the patient!

Starting with spontaneously breathing, non-paralysed patients adds extra layers of safety, since it enables the anaesthetist to also titrate drug doses according to ventilatory responses, while giving the reassurance that if anaesthesia is inadequate, the patient will be able to move, or even leave the room!

Once sufficient confidence has been gained, the N_2O can be omitted. If propofol is used alone then higher doses/target concentrations will be required. N_2O can of course be substituted for remifentanil. Bear in mind however, that it is difficult to maintain spontaneous ventilation whilst a patient receives remifentanil and propofol, so that mechanical ventilation will almost certainly be required, although this is quite easily achieved via a LMA in many patients without muscle relaxants. Eventually, with further experience and confidence, more challenging cases can be attempted, including ones where muscle relaxation is required.

4. Target-controlled infusions of opioids

As with propofol infusions, if blood targeting is used and rapid onset of analgesia is required, then the blood concentration should initially be set to a level higher than the likely therapeutic effect-site concentration. After induction of anaesthesia, the target concentrations should be adjusted according to the clinical responses of the patient. Patient movement, and increases in heart rate and blood pressure, in response to an increase in the intensity of noxious stimulus are most logically treated by increases in the level of analgesia.

When propofol/remifentanil combinations are used, it is probably best to start the propofol infusion first at induction of anaesthesia, because the effect-site remifentanil concentrations rise more rapidly than the propofol concentrations. If the remifentanil infusion is started first the patient is more likely to stop breathing before loss of consciousness, and if loss of consciousness occurs slowly, this may result in hypoxaemia while the airway is being secured, even if the patient was pre-oxygenated with 100% O_2. On some occasions it may be necessary to use bag and mask ventilation to improve oxygenation before consciousness is completely lost, and this may cause the patient distress. Anecdotal reports also suggest that chest wall rigidity associated with high doses of remifentanil is less likely if propofol is given before the remifentanil infusion is started.

It should be remembered that, as with the hypnotics, no firm recommendations can be made for target concentrations for the opioids, since pharmacokinetic and pharmacodynamic differences between patients make it essential to titrate the target concentration according to the intensity of the surgical stimulus and of course the patient response. If remifentanil is used, effect-site concentrations of the order of 4-6 ng/ml are required for adequate analgesia during laryngoscopy and tracheal intubation. Slightly lower concentrations are necessary for laryngeal mask airway insertion. During very painful operations such as laparotomy, concentrations of 6-8 ng/ml are usually necessary, whereas during cardiac surgery concentrations of the order of 10-12 ng/ml should be used. In many situations experienced anaesthetists will sometimes use higher concentrations than needed for analgesia, to maximise the hypnotic sparing effect of remifentanil.

For alfentanil, in combination with propofol, Cp50 values reported by Vuyk were: 92 ng/ml for laryngoscopy, 84 ng/ml for peritoneal incision, and 66 ng/ml for the intra-abdominal part of a laparotomy.[143] The values concord well with the experience of anaesthetists who administer alfentanil by manual bolus or infusion – the commonly used induction bolus dose of 15 µg/kg will provide a peak effect-site concentration of 85 ng/ml at ~3 mins. An infusion rate of neat alfentanil (500 µg/ml) at 10 ml/hr, gradually reducing to 5 ml/hr over 30 mins is required to maintain this concentration.

During cardiac surgery, where the hypnotic-sparing effect of the opioids will enhance cardio-stability, target concentrations in the range 150-220 ng/ml are commonly used.

5. High risk patients (Elderly, unwell, or patients with limited cardiac reserve)

Caution should always be exercised with patients who are elderly, unwell or who have limited cardiovascular reserve. Because these patients have altered pharmacokinetics (volumes of distribution, and distribution and metabolic clearance rates are often reduced when compared with fitter, younger patients), equivalent doses calculated on the basis of body weight will often result in far higher blood concentrations than would otherwise be expected. Moreover, for given blood and effect-site concentrations the hypnotics and opiates tend to produce more profound pharmacodynamic effects in the elderly and unwell, because of greater receptor sensitivity. Not only do these patients lose consciousness at lower blood and effect-site concentrations, they also will develop cardio-respiratory compromise at lower concentrations.

These differences in pharmacokinetics and pharmacodynamics in the elderly make it imperative to consider carefully the target concentrations to be used in these patients, and to titrate these according to effect even more carefully. Simpler models tend not to include age as a co-variate, and when these models are used to control a target-controlled infusion, then it is wise to use lower target concentrations for sedation and for induction and maintenance of anaesthesia.

In the very old and frail, or in patients with serious cardiac problems, it is best when inducing anaesthesia with TCI propofol, to start at very low target concentrations (e.g. 1.5 µg/ml) and to increase the target concentration in small steps (e.g. 0.5 µg/ml) every few minutes. With this approach, speed of induction is sacrificed in return for improved cardiovascular stability. In practise though, patients with cardiovascular compromise who are about to undergo cardiac surgery, typically have received a sedative pre-medication, and then a large dose of opioid during induction, and commonly lose consciousness at fairly low blood and effect-site propofol concentrations.

In frail or unwell patients not undergoing cardiac surgery, improved cardiovascular stability can be achieved by using a combination of a moderately high dose of remifentanil (eg. an infusion rate of infusion rate of ~0.25-0.3 µg/kg/min or a target concentration of 6-8 ng/ml) with a lower dose of hypnotic (eg. propofol infused at 3-5 mg/kg/hr or at a target concentration of 1.5-2.5 µg/ml). When these doses of remifentanil are used in these patients all airway reflexes are completely suppressed, so that it is often feasible to mechanically ventilate the lungs without muscle relaxations, thereby giving the anaesthetist the reassurance that if the hypnotic dose is insufficient, the patient will be able to let him know by moving (or by leaving the operating theatre in extreme circumstances!). Use of depth of anaesthesia monitors in these circumstances can also be reassuring, and may help to reduce the dose of hypnotic anaesthetic agent, reduce costs and improve cardiovascular stability.

6. Post-operative analgesia after remifentanil infusions

Commonly used target concentrations of remifentanil will prevent responses to all but the most severe of surgical stimuli, but within minutes of the infusion stopping the patient will revert from having profound analgesia to none at all. If an infusion of remifentanil is used with a hypnotic to maintain anaesthesia during a procedure that is likely to result in significant post-operative pain, then it is very important to ensure that adequate longer-acting measures have been taken to treat pain once the infusion of remifentanil has been switched off, otherwise the patient is likely to wake up in severe pain.

The options for ensuring analgesia on return of consciousness include one or more of the following: simple analgesics (e.g. paracetamol or non-steroidal anti-inflammatory drugs administered per rectum or via the intravenous route), wound infiltration, local or regional anaesthetic blocks, long-acting opioids such as morphine, or continuing the remifentanil infusion into the post-operative period. If morphine is to be used for post-operative analgesia then it is important to administer an intravenous bolus dose at least 40 minutes before the end of the anaesthetic. Munoz and colleagues administered standard doses of morphine at different intervals before the end of laparoscopic cholecystectomy in 120 adults, and found that pain scores and rescue analgesia requirements were significantly lower in those who received their morphine > 40 minutes before the end of surgery.[161]

In general, unless patients are to undergo a period of sedation and post-operative mechanical ventilation, post-operative remifentanil infusions are not practical and safe. The main problem is the narrow therapeutic index. Remifentanil has potent respiratory depressant effects – respiratory drive is reduced, and airway reflexes are obtunded – so that it is difficult to achieve a balance between adequate analgesia, and a patient who continues breathing. A solution to this problem is to give the patient some degree of control over the administration of the drug. While patient-controlled administration of remifentanil boluses has been successfully used in patients experiencing intermittent pain such as labour pains[162-164] the short-duration of action makes boluses unsuitable for post-surgical pain. A patient-maintained analgesia system, similar in concept to the patient-maintained sedation systems mentioned earlier, have been developed and used successfully under experimental conditions for control of pain during burns dressing changes,[165] and for control of pain after major spinal surgery,[166] cardiac surgery,[167,168] and orthopaedic surgery.[169] As with patient-maintained sedation these systems combine patient-controlled technology with target-controlled infusion technology. When the system is activated it starts a remifentanil or alfentanil TCI at a pre-set target concentration. After that, if the patient presses an activating button the system increases the target concentration. If he does not press the button for a period of time, then the system slowly reduces the target concentration, thereby maintaining safety.

7. Combinations of hypnotic and opioid agents

The pharmacokinetic and pharmacodynamic interactions among the anaesthetic agents have already been discussed. To reiterate, pharmacokinetic interactions may result in slightly higher concentrations of the opioid and hypnotic than expected had either agent been used alone. On the other hand, pharmacodynamic interactions result in combinations of anaesthetic agents causing far more profound clinical effects than would be expected at the same concentrations had the hypnotic agent been given alone. On their own, opioids have only minimal effects on blood pressure and cardiac output, but when combined with a hypnotic, they potentiate the detrimental cardio-respiratory effects of the hypnotic agents. Thus when hypnotics and opioids are combined, the hypnotic dose should be decreased to avoid potentially serious adverse effects such as cardiovascular instability.

7.1. Propofol and remifentanil

Moderate doses of remifentanil can halve the propofol dose requirements (see section on pharmacodynamic interactions and Table 5, p. 93). When a propofol/remifentanil combination is used the respiratory drive is significantly depressed. When used for anaesthesia, it is very difficult to reach a happy medium in which analgesia and anaesthesia are adequate, but spontaneous ventilation is maintained. Thus for anaesthesia with this combination, we would recommend using a remifentanil dose of at least 2 ng/ml (0.08 µg/kg/min) to obtund the respiratory drive and airway reflexes, and to employ mechanical ventilation of the lungs (either via an endotracheal tube or a laryngeal mask airway when this is feasable).

There are some clinical situations where there are clear benefits to using a propofol and remifentanil combination with local anaesthesia for conscious sedation. These include operations such as awake craniotomy and insertion of tension-free vaginal tape (TVT) insertion, where a combination of anxiolysis and analgesia are ideal, and the brief periods of intense stimuli can be dealt with by short-term increases in the remifentanil infusion rate. If the combination is used for conscious sedation, then extreme caution is required to avoid profound respiratory depression. Although some authors (such as Manninen et al)[170] have reported use of higher doses, based on our personal experience, for these operations we would recommend the use of target propofol concentrations of 0.5-2 µg/ml (1-4 mg/kg/hr) with target remifentanil concentrations of 0.8-1.5 ng/ml (0.03-0.06 µg/kg/min). For both agents we would recommend keeping to the lower end of the target range, with only brief increases to the higher target or infusion rate ranges.

7.2. Inhalational anaesthetic agents and remifentanil

In general the opioids have a MAC-sparing effect on the volatile anaesthetic agents. Remifentanil, sufentanil and fentanyl all have potent MAC-sparing effects on isoflurane –doses of 1.5, 0.14 and 1.67 ng/ml respectively will reduce the MAC of isoflurane by 50%.[171] For sevoflurane a similar magnitude of synergism has been shown. Albertin showed that in the presence of 60% nitrous oxide a low dose of remifentanil (1ng/ml) reduced the sevoflurane dose required to prevent a sympathetic response to incision from 2.8 to 1.1%, a 60% reduction.[172,173]

Different groups have published conflicting results on the influence of remifentanil on desflurane requirements. For example, Billard[174] found that remifentanil did not affect desflurane requirements during des/remi/N2O anaesthesia, whereas Albertin[175] found that in the presence of 60% N2O the desflurane concentration required to prevent a sympathetic response to incision decreased from 6.25% to 2.7% with 1 ng/ml and to 2.0% with 3 ng/ml remifentanil.

8. Practical precautions and pitfalls

8.1. Dedicated cannula

When administering intravenous anaesthesia, it is advisable to administer the anaesthetic agents through a dedicated intravenous cannula. The danger of administering the drugs via a cannula that is also being used for intravenous fluids is that the rate of administration depends on the flow of the fluids, and the "dead-space" in the administration set (i.e. the internal volume of administration set distal to the point where the drugs join the intravenous fluid flow). If the intravenous fluids run out, and the dead-space volume is significant, the patient may not receive any anaesthetic agent for several minutes. A more serious problem can arise if the resistance to flow through the cannula increases, and the intravenous fluids are being administered passively (under the influence of gravity). In these situations, the drug may then flow "away from the patient" towards the intravenous fluid container, and it may take many minutes before the anaesthetist notices this. In both circumstances, there is a serious risk of awareness while drug delivery is interrupted. Once the problem is recognised, and the anaesthetist has attached a new bag of intravenous fluid or relieved an obstruction, the patient will receive a bolus of the anaesthetic drugs that were occupying the dead-space volume and the fluid administration set) and if this bolus is large then adverse haemodynamic effects may result.

If it is necessary to co-administer fluids and drugs via the same cannula then it is a good idea to use a one-way valve in the fluid administration set (proximal to the point at which the drugs join the flow) to prevent the drugs from flowing the wrong way.

When a dedicated cannula or a central line is used, and it has a large bore and/or a large dead-space, then it is important to remember that at the end of the case the residual drug in the dead-space should be withdrawn, or the lines should be flushed, before the patient is returned to the post-anaesthetic care area. Failing this, if the post-anaesthesia staff are unaware of the problem and administer another drug or fluid via the same line, a significant bolus may be given with potentially serious adverse effects such as loss of consciousness and/or respiratory depression.

8.2. Administration sets

Numerous varieties of intravenous anaesthetic agent administration sets are available. For situations where two or more drugs are being infused it is best to purchase sets designed for this purpose. These sets are usually constructed of a rigid material (low compliance), have low internal volume, and have anti-syphon valves close on the pump ends of the lines. Also desirable are one-way valves in the tubing from each pump to prevent reflux of one drug towards the pump for the other, and a side port to enable co-administration of another agent or even intravenous fluids should that be necessary. Ideally the lines from the different pumps should be lightly bonded to each other for the sake of tidiness and ease of use. Ready-made sets can often be purchased for less than the cost of the individual components thereby saving money and time.

8.3. Single patient use

Current regulations stipulate that any ampoule or vial of anaesthetic agent is for single patient use. Intravenous anaesthetic agent disposables such as administration lines, three-way tapes and one-way valves are all strictly for single patient use.

8.4. Mixing two or more drugs in one syringe

With the possible exception of the addition of lignocaine to propofol to reduce pain in the arm on induction of anaesthesia, there are few situations where drug mixtures can be recommended.

While there may be anecdotal reports of success with use of hypnotic and opiate mixtures there are pitfalls associated with this practise. The first is that when two drugs are mixed the mixture is legally regarded as a new, unlicensed drug, for which the anaesthetist assumes all liability. The second is that the agents may not be pharmaceutically compatible – the mixture may not be stable, one or both drugs may precipitate etc. Finally, it is very unlikely that any two anaesthetic agents will have identical pharmacokinetic properties. Thus if for example a target-controlled infusion device is used, in an attempt to provide a target concentration of one component of the mixture, problems may arise when the target is increased or decreased. On an increase, the bolus dose of the second drug may be very large, whereas, when the target is decreased, and the infusion stops for a period of time, if the second drug is metabolised at a greater rate than the first, then the blood and effect-site concentrations of the second drug may fall to excessively low levels.

8.5. Drug concentrations

In general it is good practise where possible, to always use the same concentrations of drugs for all patients, whether administering boluses or infusions manually, or administering target-controlled infusions. There are several potential problems with using different concentrations. The first is the likelihood of calculation errors. When an anaesthetist calculates the volume of a bolus, or the rate of an infusion, errors are more likely if an unfamiliar concentration is used, particularly when the anaesthetist has to make the calculation under pressure, or when the concentration is different for different patients on an operating schedule.

The second and third reasons concern changing the concentrations of drugs being administered by infusion during the conduct of a case. When administering any infusion, there is always an amount of "deadspace" in the administration set and in the intravenous cannula. The second reason for not changing concentrations is that after a change, there is a period of time during which the deadspace contains a more or less concentrated solution of the drug, and this may cause blood concentrations to fall or rise before the new solution reaches the vascular tree. This applies to manually controlled and target-controlled infusions and is particularly pertinent when drugs are administered via central venous cannulae, which may have internal volumes of up to 2 ml.

With the Diprifusor-containing generation of TCI propofol pumps, it was possible to safely change the concentration of propofol being used during the conduct of a case, because the pumps were able to recognise which concentration the pre-filled syringe in use contained (ie. 1 or 2% propofol). No other pumps, including the new open-TCI pumps, have this facility to recognise the type or concentration of the drug that is loaded in the syringe. More importantly, none of the currently available pumps have the facility for the user to inform the pump that the concentration has been changed during the conduct of the case. If a syringe is replaced by another containing a greater or lesser concentration than the system assumes to be in use, increasingly large prediction errors in the blood and effect-site concentrations will occur, and these cannot be corrected by simply increasing or decreasing the target concentration.

8.6. Concentrated drug solutions, and low target concentrations and/or small patients

Most modern infusion pumps used in the operating theatres are syringe drivers. In essence, the system recognises the diameter of the syringe, and for a given infusion rate calculates the distance that the plunger has to be pushed in per unit of time to infuse at that rate (this distance is inversely proportional to the square of the radius of the syringe). The distance the plunger should be displaced over a unit of time is then "translated" into an angular velocity or a quantity of completed rotations per unit of time of the driving motor, and the slower the angular rotation, the less accurate the rate of infusion becomes over small units of time. These and other factors limit the precision of most pumps to 0.1 ml/hr.

During target-controlled infusions the system keeps a track of the total volume infused in each period of time, by monitoring the number of rotations of the motor. At the end of each 10 sec epoch the system calculates the difference between the dose that should have been administered and what was administered, and makes an allowance to correct for any error during the following epoch – this is why the infusion rate is often seen to "oscillate" between two different infusion rates while the target concentration is kept constant. The slower the infusion rate the greater the relative size of these oscillations. If a concentrated drug solution is used, then small errors in infusion rate during an epoch may result in larger (but still generally clinically insignificant) oscillating errors in the blood concentration.

When the required infusion rate is small (as with low target concentrations or small patients), and a concentrated drug solution is used, it is wise to select the smallest syringe size practical, to maximise the displacement of the syringe plunger required. It is also important to use good quality syringes. When the infusion rate and the angular rotation of the motor are slow, the quality of the syringe becomes very important. If the rubber stopper is very compressible, or the lubricant between the stopper and the side walls of the syringe is poorly or unevenly applied, then the stopper may move in small steps rather than continuously, in effect administering a series of boluses rather than an infusion. Use of a good quality small syringe will thus improve the accuracy and stability of the infusion rate.

V. The future

In recent years, competition from generic versions of propofol and some of the older opioid analgesics, has caused significant reductions in the costs of these drugs. As more anaesthetists gain access to TCI systems for these agents, it is likely that the popularity and frequency of use of intravenous anaesthesia in general, and target controlled infusions in particular, will increase. Now that TIVA has become established in adult practise it is likely they it will increasingly be used in children, who will also be able to enjoy the benefits of TIVA and TCI.

1. New, improved models

Most models in use at the present work best for healthy adults, but do not apply to, or perform poorly when used for young, elderly or unwell patients. Although more sophisticated models for use in special populations (young, elderly) have been published, few studies have validated the predictive performance of TCI systems in these groups. This is likely to change with time. We might see models that apply to these specific groups, or general models that can take into account more of the co-variates such as age, that are responsible for the inter-patient pharmacokinetic variability. New models, or improvements to current models are likely to be associated with more accurate control of targeted blood and effect-site drug concentrations.

The current trend of an increasing incidence of obesity is likely to be maintained. Further research into the pharmacokinetics of anaesthetic drugs in the obese is required, as are studies specifically investigating the performance of the current models in the obese. Hopefully a better formula for lean body mass will be found, and will provide meaningful and useful values for a broader range of patients. If such a new formula is developed and accepted, then the current models using lean body mass may require revision.

2. New drugs

No new volatile anaesthetic agents have been discovered within the last few decades. In the future, it is likely that there will be pressure from governments and regulatory authorities to reduce the usage of agents with harmful environmental effects, and this might cause a decline in the use of volatile anaesthetic agents, which would in turn stimulate the development and use of newer, safe intravenous agents.

None of the currently available intravenous anaesthetic agents is perfect. Hopefully new, improved drugs with improved pharmacokinetic and pharmacodynamic profiles will be discovered and introduced. Perhaps one day we will have short-acting agents that cause anxiolysis without sedation and respiratory depression, analgesics that don't cause nausea and vomiting and hypnotics that don't cause pain on injection and cardio-respiratory compromise.

The results of clinical trials of a new esterase-metabolised hypnotic agent, THRX 198661, are eagerly awaited. If safe and effective for use in humans this drug should be eminently suitable for use by TCI, and should offer a similar speed of onset and recovery to that of remifentanil.

3. Patient-controlled TCI systems

Patient-controlled TCI systems, when used for sedation and analgesia, have been popular[172] with patients, surgeons and anaesthetists, and bring potential improvements in safety and patient satisfaction. It is likely that patient-control functionality will be added to commercially available TCI pumps in the not-too-distant future.

4. Closed loop control of anaesthesia

Auditory evoked potentials and the Bispectral Index have been used by computerised systems to automatically control infusions of propofol for sedation[176,177] and general anaesthesia.[178-181] These systems have the potential to provide more accurate control of anaesthesia. For optimal function closed loop systems require control variables that accurately reflect the process being controlled. Progress with our understanding of the process of anaesthesia, coupled with improved measures of anaesthetic depth could see increased use of computer control of anaesthesia.

VI. Case studies

Seven cases are presented here to give an idea of the range of concentrations required for different cases, and a flavour of the possibilities of use of intravenous anaesthesia. They should not be used as a fixed recipe for using TIVA or TCI, because each patient is different and the dose of any drug should always be titrated to individual requirements.

For each case a description of the case is presented first followed by a figure showing haemodynamic data, estimated blood and effect-site hypnotic and opiate concentrations and a table showing the timing of drug administration and other events. Haemodynamic data, recorded manually, are shown in the top panel for each case. Heart rate data are represented by diamonds, and the arterial blood pressure by vertical bars (the upper limits of which represents the systolic arterial pressure and the lower limits the diastolic pressure). For some of the cases an EEG (electroencephalogram) based measure of anaesthetic depth was recorded and is also shown. These include the Bispectral Index (BIS), auditory evoked potential index (AEPI), median frequency (MF) and spectral edge frequency (SEF).

Case 1: Conscious sedation for insertion of tension-free vaginal tape

History:

The patient was a 45 year old female, who suffered from stress incontinence. Her obstetric history consisted of 4 natural vaginal deliveries. She was a non-smoker and had no other significant past medical history. Although very anxious, she preferred to have the procedure performed under a combination of local anaesthesia and conscious sedation, rather than general anaesthesia.

Surgical procedure:
Insertion of tension-free vaginal tape

Anaesthetic management:
While routine physiological monitoring was commenced, an intravenous cannula was inserted, prophylactic antibiotics were administered and a crystalloid infusion containing 75 mg diclofenac was commenced. A blood targeted propofol infusion (using the Marsh model) was started (Event 1). In order to hasten the increase in the effect-site concentration (and hence the onset of clinical effect), the blood target was initially set to 2 µg/ml, but once

that target concentration was attained the target was reduced to 1 µg/ml. At the same time a 0.5 µg/kg bolus of remifentanil was administered, followed by an infusion at 0.03 µg/kg/min. Within 10 minutes the patient was calm and comfortable, and the surgical team was invited to commence preparations for the operation. From this point until the end of the operation oxygen was administered via a face mask at 4 L/min.

Just before local anaesthetic infiltration the target propofol concentration was increased to 1.2 µg/ml and a second 0.5 µg/kg remifentanil bolus was administered. The surgeon infiltrated the operative sites (vulva, retro-pubic area and suprapubic area) with 50 ml of a 0.1% levo-bupivacaine and 1:100 000 adrenaline mixture (Event 2), and commenced the operation. After a further 30 min the surgeon was ready to insert the tapes (this requires the use of very large curved needles). Just prior to tape insertion a third 0.5 µg/kg remifentanil bolus was given (Event 3).

Ten minutes later the procedure was completed, and all infusions were stopped (Event 4). The patient had remained conscious (responsive to voice) throughout the procedure.

Post-operative course:

The patient spent 30 min in the recovery room (post-anaesthesia care unit), before being transferred to her ward, where she spent an uneventful night before being discharged home.

Case 1: Conscious sedation for insertion of tension-free vaginal tape. The top panel shows the haemodynamic data, the middle panel the estimated blood and effect-site propofol and remifentanil concentrations, while the lower panel shows the timing of drug administration and other events

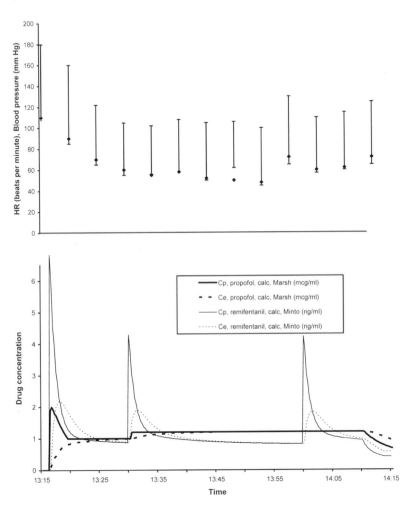

Case 2: Examination under anaesthesia, sigmoidoscopy

History:

The patient was a 21 old male, who had a history of bleeding per rectum. He smoked 20 cigarettes per day, and consumed 21 units of alcohol per week.

Surgical procedure:

Examination under anaesthesia, sigmoidoscopy

Anaesthetic management:

While routine physiological monitoring was commenced and baseline measurements were being taken, an intravenous cannula was inserted and BIS electrodes (Aspect Medical Systems, Newton, USA) were applied to the forehead. The electrodes were then connected to an A-2000 BIS monitor (Aspect Medical Systems, Newton, USA). A 75 µg bolus of fentanyl was administered, and a blood targeted propofol infusion (Marsh model) was started (Event 1) with an initial target concentration of 6 µg/ml. After that the target blood propofol concentration was increased by 0.5 µg/ml every 30 sec until loss of consciousness (Event 2). A laryngeal mask airway was inserted (Event 3), via which the patient breathed 40% oxygen in air. The patient was placed in the lithotomy position.

Just before the surgeon commenced the procedure (Event 4) a further 25 µg bolus of fentanyl was administered. Towards the end of the surgical procedure the target propofol concentration was reduced to 4 µg/ml, and once the procedure was finished (Event 5) the target was set to zero. The patient regained consciousness soon after (at a BIS of 86), the laryngeal mask airway was removed and the patient was transferred to the recovery room.

Post-operative course:

The patient spent 15 min in the recovery room, and was discharged home after an uneventful 3 hour stay on the day surgery ward.

Case 2: General anaesthesia for examination under anaesthesia and sigmoidoscopy. The top panel shows the haemodynamic data, the middle panel the estimated blood and effect-site propofol and fentanyl concentrations, while the lower panel shows the timing of drug administration and other events

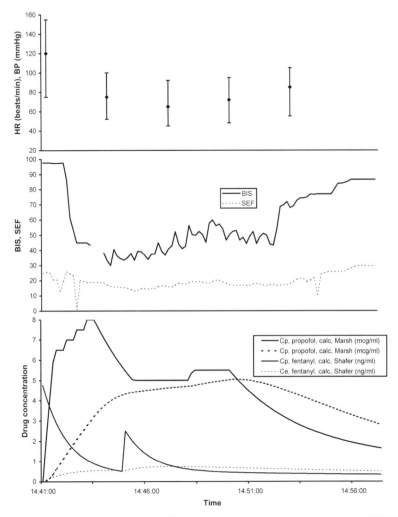

Propofol trgt (µg/ml)	6-----7--8--5------------------------5.2----------4----0				
Fentanyl (µg)	75	25			
Events	1	2, 3	4	5	6

Case 3: Inguinal hernia repair

History:

The patient was a 55 year old male, who smoked 30 cigarettes per day, had a chronic cough and a left inguinal hernia.

Surgical procedure:

Inguinal hernia repair (mesh)

Anaesthetic management:

While routine physiological monitoring was commenced and baseline measurements were being taken, an intravenous cannula was inserted and Zipprep electrodes (Aspect Medical Systems, Newton, USA) were applied to the forehead and mastoid process. The electrodes were connected to a custom-developed Auditory Evoked Potential system that calculated the Auditory Evoked Potential Index (AEPI). The auditory stimulus was applied via small earplugs.

Target-controlled infusions of propofol and remifentanil were started at target concentrations of 6 µg/ml and 6 ng/ml respectively (Event 1). After loss of consciousness (eyelash reflex) (Event 2) the propofol target concentration was reduced to 4 µg/ml, and a laryngeal mask airway was inserted soon afterwards (Event 3) and the patients lungs were mechanically ventilated with 40% oxygen in air. The propofol target concentration was reduced to 2.5 µg/ml, and an ilio-inguinal block was performed with 10 ml of 0.5% bupivacaine. An intravenous infusion of 1000 ml of compound sodium lactate, also containing 75 mg diclofenac, was commenced.

Cefuroxime 1.5 g was administered as prophylaxis against infection of the prosthetic material used in the repair, and the surgeon started the operation (event 4). During the operation 5 mg intravenous morphine was given. As the surgeon began the final skin sutures, the target propofol and remifentanil concentrations were reduced to 2.2 µg/ml and 3 ng/ml respectively. At the end of the operation (event 5) the infusions were switched off, and the patient regained consciousness soon after (event 6).

Post-operative course:

The patient spent 30 min in the recovery room, and was discharged home after an uneventful 4 hour stay on the day surgery ward.

Case 3: Inguinal hernia repair. From top to bottom the panels show: haemodynamic data, Auditory Evoked Potential Index, the estimated propofol and remifentanil concentrations, and timing of drug administration and other events

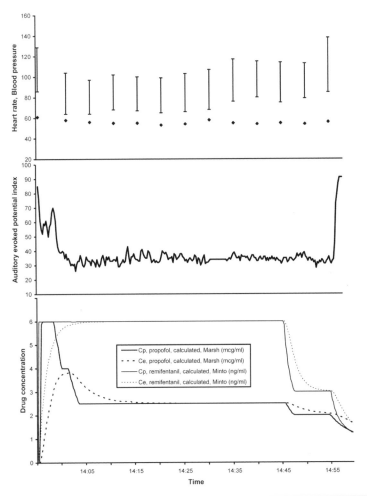

Propofol target (μg/ml)	6—4—2.5--0
Remi. target (ng/ml)	6--3---------0
Bupivacaine	10 ml 0.5% (ilio-inguinal block)
Diclofenac	75 mg (in 1000 ml compound sodium lactate)--------------------
Morphine (mg)	5 mg
Events	1,2,3, 4, 5, 6

Case 4: Total hip replacement under combined general and regional anaesthesia (using TCI propofol and epidural local anaesthetic boluses)

History:

The patient was a 69 year old female, who was overweight and had a history of osteoarthritis.

Surgical procedure:

Total hip replacement.

Anaesthetic management:

Routine physiological monitoring was commenced and baseline measurements recorded. Two intravenous cannula were inserted: a 22G for intravenous drug administration, and a 16G for intravenous fluid administration. An infusion of a crystalloid solution was started immediately. Later in the case 1000ml of a synthetic colloid solution was also administered.

Intravenous cefuroxime 1.5g was given for surgical prophylaxis, and a 3mg bolus of midazolam for anxiolysis. After local anaesthetic infiltration of the skin, with the patient in the sitting position, a high lumbar epidural catheter was inserted. A test dose of 3 ml 0.5% bupivacaine was administered into the epidural space, followed by a bolus of 7 ml of 0.5% bupivacaine. After 20 min the patient had a sensory level (to cold sensation) at T10.

Zipprep electrodes (Aspect Medical Systems, Newton, USA) were applied in a bipolar montage (FP1 – AT1, FP2 – AT2, reference FPZ), and connected to an A-1000 monitor (Aspect Medical Systems, Newton, USA, software version 3.22) from which the Bispectral Index, SEF and MF were continuously recorded. Using an estimate of the ideal body mass, a blood concentration targeted infusion of propofol (Marsh model) was started at an initial target of 4 µg/ml (event 1). The patient soon lost consciousness (loss of eyelash reflex, event 2), and the target propofol concentration was reduced to 2 µg/ml. A laryngeal mask airway was inserted (event 3) through which the patient spontaneously breathed 40% oxygen in air.

Just before the first surgical incision the target concentration was increased to 3 µg/ml. The BIS rose after the incision (event 4), but soon decreased, and so the target was reduced to 2.2 µg/ml and later to 2 µg/ml. During the operation the patient had two brief episodes of arousal (movement associated with an increase in the BIS). The first was during some vigorous hammering (event 5) and the second during manipulation of the limb to locate the prosthetic joint (event 6). In both cases the depth of anaesthesia was increased by temporary increases in the target propofol concentration. After the second episode a 10 ml epidural bolus of 0.25% bupivacaine was administered.

During final manipulation of the hip the BIS rose, and so the target propofol concentration was again increased until just before the end of the operation when it was reduced to 2 µg/ml, before being switched to zero when the final skin suture was in place (event 7). The patient regained consciousness soon after (event 8).

Post-operative course:

The patient spent 2 hours in the recovery room, during which time simple oral analgesics were administered, an epidural infusion containing 0.1% bupivacaine and clonidine 0.6 ng/ml was started (and continued for 3 days after which the catheter was removed). The post-operative course was uncomplicated and the patient was discharged home on the 5th post-operative day.

Case 4: Combined general and regional anaesthesia for total hip replacement. From top to bottom the panels show: haemodynamic data, EEG data (BIS, SEF and MF), the estimated propofol concentrations, and timing of drug administration and other events

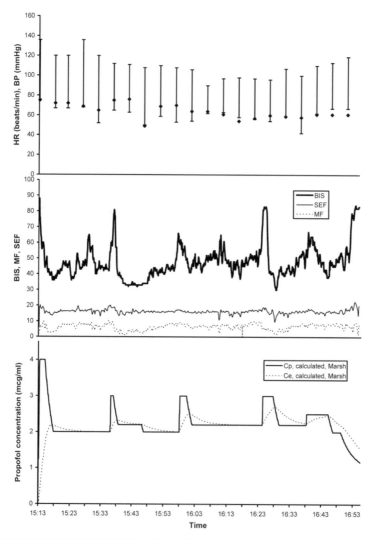

Midazolam	3 mg
Propofol target (μg/ml)	4-2--------------3-2.2---2--------3-2.2----------------3- 2.2-----2.5---2-0
Bupivacaine	10 ml 0.25%
Ketorolac	10 mg 20 mg
Cefuroxime	1.5 g
Events	1,2, 3, 4, 5, 6, 7, 8

Case 5: Clipping of peri-callosal aneurysm using effect-site targeted propofol (Schnider model) and remifentanil infusions (Minto model)

History:

The patient was a 48 year old female, who smoked 20 cigarettes per day, and had a 10 day history of headache, and paraesthesia in her face, arms and trunk. Angiography demonstrated the cause to be a peri-callosal cerebral aneurysm.

Surgical procedure:

Craniotomy, clipping of peri-callosal aneurysm

Anaesthetic management:

Routine non-invasive physiological monitoring was commenced and baseline measurements recorded. After local anaesthetic infiltration of the skin a 14G intravenous cannula was inserted, and an infusion of 1000 ml of a crystalloid solution commenced. Later in the case the intravenous fluids administered comprised 250 ml of 20% mannitol, a further 1000 ml of crystalloid and 1000 ml of a synthetic colloid solution. Antibiotic prophylaxis comprised flucloxacillin 1g and gentamycin 120 mg.

After the patient had breathed 100% oxygen for 3 mins, anaesthetic induction was commenced (event 1) with effect-site targeted infusions of propofol (Schnider model) and remifentanil (Minto model), at target concentrations of 6 µg/ml and 8 ng/ml respectively. The patient lost consciousness 2 min later (event 2), after which the muscle relaxant (pancuronium) was administered. Two minutes later endotracheal intubation was performed (event 3), and the target concentrations were reduced to 3 µg/ml and 6 ng/ml respectively. Central venous access was secured, and a radial artery catheter and a urinary catheter were inserted. After application of the scalp pins of the Mayfield head holder (event 4), the target propofol concentration was reduced to 2.2 µg/ml.

Just before the first skin incision (event 5), while a weak mixture of lignocaine and epinephrine were infiltrated into the scalp, the target propofol concentration was increased to 2.5 µg/ml. The systolic arterial pressure later drifted below 100 mmHg, requiring one small dose of metaraminol, and a reduction of the target propofol concentration.

A permanent clip was applied (event 6) without the need for a temporary clip. Morphine 5 mg was administered for post-operative analgesia. When the skin sutures were started (event 7) the target remifentanil concentration was reduced to 5 ng/ml, and after the Mayfield pins were removed (event 8) both target concentrations were reduced to zero. The patient recovered consciousness within 5 minutes (event 9).

Post-operative course:

The patient spent an hour in the recovery room during which time she required 1 g of intravenous paracetamol and a further 3mg of intravenous morphine for pain relief. She made an uneventful recovery and was discharged home on the 4th postoperative day.

Case 5: *Clipping of peri-callosal aneurysm using effect-site targeted propofol (Schnider model) and remifentanil infusions (Minto model). From top to bottom the panels show: haemodynamic data, the estimated blood and effect-site propofol and remifentanil concentrations, the timing of drug administration and other events*

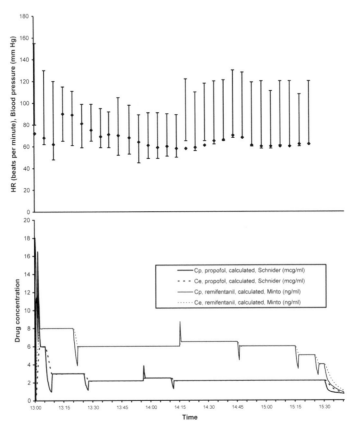

Propofol target (µg/ml)	6,4,3-----2.2-------------2.5-----2.2---------------------------------------0
Remif. target (ng/ml)	8-------6-------------------------6.5--------------6---------------5---4--0
Pancuronium (mg)	8
Metaraminol (mg)	0.5
Morphine (mg)	5
Events	1,2,3, 4, 5, 6, 7, 8, 9

Case 6: Excision of skin lesion under general anaesthesia using blood concentration targeted infusions of propofol (Marsh model) and alfentanil (Maitre model)

History:

The patient was a 35 year old male, who had a large skin lesion that required excision biopsy.

Surgical procedure:

Excision of skin lesion

Anaesthetic management:

While routine physiological monitoring was commenced, an intravenous cannula was inserted and BIS electrodes (Aspect Medical Systems, Newton, USA) were applied to the forehead. The electrodes were connected to an A-2000 BIS monitor (Aspect Medical Systems, Newton, USA), which calculated the BIS and SEF, which were recorded electronically. Physiological measurements were made and recorded every 5 min thereafter.

Intravenous anaesthetic induction was commenced (event 1) using blood targeted infusions of propofol (Marsh model) and alfentanil (Maitre model). The initial target concentrations were 6 µg/ml and 80 ng/ml, respectively. At loss of consciousness, defined as loss of eyelash reflex (event 2), the target propofol concentration was reduced to 4 µg/ml. Following laryngeal mask insertion (event 3) the alfentanil target concentration was reduced to 50ng/ml, and an infusion of 1000 ml crystalloid solution, containing 75 mg of diclofenac was commenced. The lungs of the patient were mechanically ventilated with 40% oxygen in air, via the laryngeal mask airway.

The surgeon prepared the patient and then infiltrated the skin surrounding the lesion with 10 ml of 0.5% bupivacaine before making his first skin incision (event 4). When he began the final skin sutures (event 5) the alfentanil target concentration was set to zero and the propofol target reduced to 2.5 µg/ml. When the skin sutures were completed (event 6) the propofol target concentration was set to zero. After 3 min the patient regained consciousness and began to breathe spontaneously (event 7).

Post-operative course:

The patient spent 30 min in the recovery room, before being transferred to the general ward, where he was ready for discharge home within two hours. He made an uneventful recovery.

Case 6: *Excision of skin lesion under general anaesthesia.*

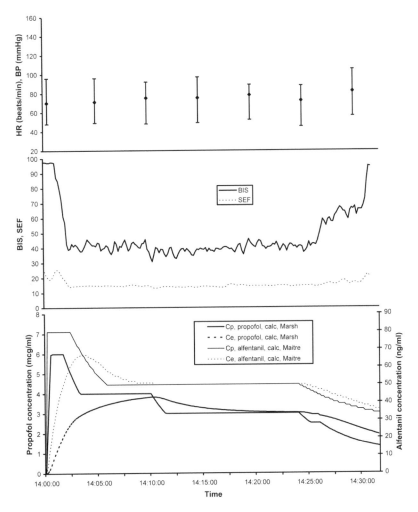

Propofol target (µg/ml)	6--4----------------------3------------------------------------2.5---0
Alfentanil target (ng/ml)	80-----50---0
Diclofenac (mg)	75 (in 1000 ml crystalloid solution) ----------
Events	1, 2, 3, 4, 5, 6, 7

Case 7: Laparotomy for partial bowel resection and reconstruction of ureter

History:

The patient was a 42 year old woman with history of severe endometriosis resulting in multiple adhesions of the intestinal structures. Recently, she had developed a colo-vesical fistula.

Surgical procedure:

Laparotomy

Anaesthetic management:

While routine physiological monitoring was commenced, an intravenous cannula was inserted and BIS electrodes (Aspect Medical Systems, Newton, USA) were applied to the forehead. The electrodes were connected to an A-2000 BIS monitor (Aspect Medical Systems, Newton, USA). Physiological measurements (heart rate, non invasive blood pressure, SpO_2, capnography, ECG, temperature) were made and recorded every 5 min thereafter. After pre-oxygenation, sufentanil effect compartment controlled TCI using the Gepts model was commenced at a target concentration of 0.3 ng/ml. Two minutes later, anaesthesia was induced with a slopw bolus of propofol 1% (1.5 mg/kg). After loss of consciousness, a bolus of rocuronium 0.6 mg/kg was given to facilitate tracheal intubation. After intubation, sevoflurane was started and titrated to maintain a BIS between 40 and 50. The patients' lungs were ventilated using IPPV to maintain normocapnia. A heating system was used to maintain normothermia, and a urinary catheter was inserted to monitor urine output. Sufentanil target concentration was titrated to maintain stable haemodynimics. A central venous line was inserted in the internal jugular vein to administer fluids and measure central venous pressure (CVP). Prophylactic antibiotic therapy was given. During the case, intermittent bolus doses of rocuronium were given when required. Details are plotted in the figure.

Forty-five minutes before the predicted end of surgery the sufentanil infusion was stopped. Intravenous paracetamol (1g) and morphine 0.15 mg/kg were given to provide postoperative pain relief. During skin closure (when the effect-site sufentanil concentration was 0.1 ng/ml) the patient started breathing spontaneously. After skin closure, sevoflurane was stopped and the endotracheal tube was removed after return of consciousness.

Post-operative recovery:

The patient was transferred to the post-operative recovery room, where a morphine intravenous PCA system was connected. The patient remained in the PACU for 24 hours and returned to the ward for further recovery. The post-operative phase was uneventful.

Case 7: Laparotomy for partial bowel resection and reconstruction of ureter

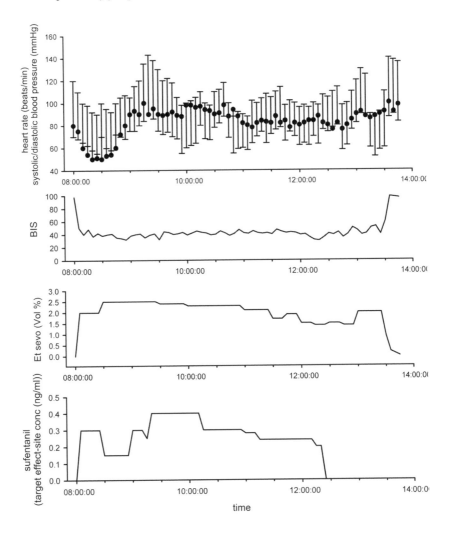

Table 1: Adult propofol models

	Marsh[42]		Schnider[45]	
	General model	70 kg	General model (LBM calculated using weight, height, gender)	70 kg, male height 170 cm
V1	0.228 L/kg	15.9 L	4.27 L	4.27 L
V2	0.463 L/kg	32.4 L	$18.9 - 0.391 \times (age - 53)$ L	24.0 L
V3	2.893 L/kg	202.0 L	238 L	238 L
K_{10} (min^{-1})	0.119	0.119	$0.443 + 0.0107 \times (weight - 77) - 0.0159 \times (LBM - 59) + 0.0062 \times (height - 177)$	0.384
K_{12} (min^{-1})	0.112	0.112	$0.302 - 0.0056 \times (age - 53)$	0.375
K_{13} (min^{-1})	0.042	0.042	0.196	0.196
K_{21} (min^{-1})	0.055	0.055	$[1.29 - 0.024 \times (age - 53)] / [18.9 - 0.391 \times (age - 53)]$	0.067
K_{31} (min^{-1})	0.0033	0.0033	0.0035	0.004
K_{e0} (min^{-1})	0.26[123]	0.26	0.456	0.456
TTPE (min)	4.5[124]	4.5	1.69	1.69

Table 2: Paediatric propofol models

	Paedfusor[49]†		Kataria[48]	
	Model	20 kg patient	Model	20 kg patient
V1	0.458 L/kg	9.2 L	0.52 L/kg	10.4 L
V2	1.34 L/kg	26.8 L	1.0 L/kg	20 L
V3	8.20 L/kg	163.9 L	8.2 L/kg	164 L
K_{10} (min^{-1})	$70 \times \text{Weight}^{-0.3}/458.4$	0.062	0.066	0.066
K_{12} (min^{-1})	0.12	0.12	0.113	0.113
K_{13} (min^{-1})	0.034	0.034	0.051	0.051
K_{21} (min^{-1})	0.041	0.041	0.059	0.059
K_{31} (min^{-1})	0.0019	0.0019	0.0032	0.0032

†. This model applies to children < 16 years old

Table 3: Other models

	Remifentanil (Minto)[53]	Sufentanil (Bovill)[56]	Sufentanil (Gepts)[55]	Alfentanil (Maitre)[63]	Fentanyl (Shafer)[28]
V_c (L)	$5.1 - 0.0201 \times (age - 40) + 0.072 \times (LBM - 55)$	0.164 L/kg	14.3	Male: 0.111 L/kg Female: 1.15×0.111 L/kg	6.09
V2 (L)	$9.82 - 0.0811 \times (age - 40) + 0.108 \times (LBM - 55)$	0.359 L/kg	63.4	12.0	28.1
V3 (L)	5.42	1.263 L/kg	251.9	10.5	228
K_{10} (min^{-1})	$[(2.6 - 0.0162 \times (age - 40) + 0.0191 \times (LBM - 55)] / V_c$	0.089	0.0645	Age <= 40 years: $0.356 / V_c$ Age < 40: $0.356 - [0.00269 \times (age - 40)] / V_c$	0.083
K_{12} (min^{-1})	$[(2.05 - 0.0301 \times (age - 40)] / V_c$	0.35	0.1086	0.104	0.4713
K_{13} (min^{-1})	$[0.076 - 0.00113 \times (age - 40)] / V_c$	0.077	0.0229	0.017	0.22496
K_{21} (min^{-1})	$K_{12} \times V_c / V2$	0.16	0.0245	0.067	0.1021
K_{31} (min^{-1})	$K13 \times V_c / V3$	0.01	0.0013	Age <= 40 years: 0.0126 Age > 40: $0.0126 - 0.000113 \times (age - 40)$	0.00601
K_{eo} (min^{-1})	$0.595 - 0.007 \times (age - 40)$	0.12	0.112	0.77 ([125])	0.147 ([125])

Table 4: Predictive performance of commonly used pharmacokinetic models

Drug	Propofol			Remifentanil	Sufentanil		Alfentanil
Model	Marsh[42]	Swinhoe[99]	Paedfusor[49] Absalom[49]	Minto[53] Mertens[102]	Gepts[55]	Barvais[103]	Maitre[63] Maitre[63]
Investigating author	Coetzee[98]						
MDPE (%)	−7.0	16.2	4.1	−15	−22.9		−7.9
MDAPE (%)	18.2	24.1	9.7	20	29.0		22.3
Wobble (%)	10.0	21.9	8.3	16			
Divergence (%)	6.5	−7.6	-	5			

Table 5: *Propofol/opioid combinations estimated by Vuyk et al to be associated with the fastest recovery from anaesthesia. $C_{optimal}$ represents combinations associated with a 50% probability of a response to surgical stimuli; $C_{awakening}$ concentrations represent the estimated concentrations at which consciousness will be regained and Times to awakening represent the estimated time from termination of the infusion to return of consciousness in 50% of patients. (From Vuyk[157])*

Infusion duration (min)		Propofol/alfentanil (µg/ml; ng/ml)	Propofol/sufentanil (µg/ml; ng/ml)	Propofol/remifentanil (µg/ml; ng/ml)
15	$C_{optimal}$	3.25 / 99.3	3.57 / 0.17	2.57 / 4.70
	$C_{awakening}$	1.69 / 65.0	1.70 / 0.10	1.83 / 1.93
	Time to awakening (min)	8.2	9.4	5.1
60	$C_{optimal}$	3.38 / 89.7	3.34 / 0.14	2.51 / 4.78
	$C_{awakening}$	1.70 / 64.9	1.70 / 0.10	1.83 / 1.93
	Time to awakening (min)	12.2	11.9	6.1
300	$C_{optimal}$	3.40 / 88.9	3.37 / 0.14	2.51 / 4.78
	$C_{awakening}$	1.70 / 64.9	1.70 / 0.10	1.86 / 1.88
	Time to awakening (min)	16.0	15.6	6.7

References

1. Lee JA: History of anaesthesia, Lee's Synopsis of Anaesthesia, 11th Edition. Edited by Atkinson RS, Rushman GB, Davies NJH. London, Butterworth Heinemann, 1996, pp 875-915
2. Absalom A, Pledger D, Kong A: Adrenocortical function in critically ill patients 24 h after a single dose of etomidate. Anaesthesia 1999; 54: 861-7
3. Doze VA, Shafer A, White PF: Propofol-nitrous oxide versus thiopental-isoflurane-nitrous oxide for general anesthesia. Anesthesiology 1988; 69: 63-71
4. Lim BL, Low TC: Total intravenous anaesthesia versus inhalational anaesthesia for dental day surgery. Anaesth Intensive Care 1992; 20: 475-8
5. Suttner S, Boldt J, Schmidt C, Piper S, Kulme B: Cost analysis of target-controlled infusion-based anesthesia compared with standard anesthesia regimens. Anesthesia and Analgesia 1999; 88: 77-82
6. Borgeat A, Wilder-Smith OH, Saiah M, Rifat K: Subhypnotic doses of propofol possess direct antiemetic properties. Anesth Analg 1992; 74: 539-41
7. Eriksson H, Korttila K: Recovery profile after desflurane with or without ondansetron compared with propofol in patients undergoing outpatient gynecological laparoscopy. Anesth Analg 1996; 82: 533-8
8. Hartung J: Twenty-four of twenty-seven studies show a greater incidence of emesis associated with nitrous oxide than with alternative anesthetics. Anesth Analg 1996; 83: 114-6
9. Raeder J, Gupta A, Pedersen FM: Recovery characteristics of sevoflurane- or propofol-based anaesthesia for day-care surgery. Acta Anaesthesiol Scand 1997; 41: 988-94
10. James MF: Nitrous oxide: still useful in the year 2000? Curr Opin Anaesthesiol 1999; 12: 461-6
11. Sukhani R, Lurie J, Jabamoni R: Propofol for ambulatory gynecologic laparoscopy: does omission of nitrous oxide alter postoperative emetic sequelae and recovery? Anesth Analg 1994; 78: 831-5
12. Smith I, Terhoeve PA, Hennart D, Feiss P, Harmer M, Pourriat JL, Johnson IA: A multicentre comparison of the costs of anaesthesia with sevoflurane or propofol. Br J Anaesth 1999; 83: 564-70
13. Lee L, Harrison LM, Mechelli A: A report of the functional connectivity workshop, Dusseldorf 2002. Neuroimage 2003; 19: 457-65
14. Hornuss C, Praun S, Villinger J, Dornauer A, Moehnle P, Dolch M, Weninger E, Chouker A, Feil C, Briegel J, Thiel M, Schelling G: Real-time monitoring of propofol in expired air in humans undergoing total intravenous anesthesia. Anesthesiology 2007; 106: 665-74
15. Kruger-Thiemer E: Continuous intravenous infusion and multicompartment accumulation. Eur J Pharmacol 1968; 4: 317-24

16. Vaughan DP, Tucker GT: General theory for rapidly establishing steady state drug concentrations using two consecutive constant rate intravenous infusions. Eur J Clin Pharmacol 1975; 9: 235-8
17. Vaughan DP, Tucker GT: General derivation of the ideal intravenous drug input required to achieve and maintain a constant plasma drug concentration. Theoretical application to lignocaine therapy. Eur.J.Clin.Pharmacol. 1976; 10: 433-440
18. Schwilden H: A general method for calculating the dosage scheme in linear pharmacokinetics. Eur J Clin Pharmacol 1981; 20: 379-86
19. Crankshaw DP, Boyd MD, Bjorksten AR: Plasma drug efflux – a new approach to optimization of drug infusion for constant blood concentration of thiopental and methohexital. Anesthesiology 1987; 67: 32-41
20. Shafer SL, Siegel LC, Cooke JE, Scott JC: Testing computer-controlled infusion pumps by simulation. Anesthesiology 1988; 68: 261-6
21. Tavernier A, Coussaert E, D'Hollander A, Cantraine F: Model-based pharmacokinetic regulation in computer-assisted anesthesia an interactive system: CARIN. Acta Anaesthesiol.Belg. 1987; 38: 63-68
22. Alvis JM, Reves JG, Govier AV, Menkhaus PG, Henling CE, Spain JA, Bradley E: Computer-assisted continuous infusions of fentanyl during cardiac anesthesia: comparison with a manual method. Anesthesiology 1985; 63: 41-49
23. Jacobs JR: Algorithm for optimal linear model-based control with application to pharmacokinetic model-driven drug delivery. IEEE Trans Biomed Eng 1990; 37: 107-9
24. Jacobs JR, Williams EA: Algorithm to control "effect compartment" drug concentrations in pharmacokinetic model-driven drug delivery. IEEE Trans Biomed Eng 1993; 40: 993-9
25. Shafer SL, Gregg KM: Algorithms to rapidly achieve and maintain stable drug concentrations at the site of drug effect with a computer-controlled infusion pump. J Pharmacokinet Biopharm 1992; 20: 147-69
26. Ausems ME, Stanski DR, Hug CC: An evaluation of the accuracy of pharmacokinetic data for the computer assisted infusion of alfentanil. Br J Anaesth 1985; 57: 1217-1225
27. Glass PS, Jacobs JR, Smith LR, Ginsberg B, Quill TJ, Bai SA, Reves JG: Pharmacokinetic model-driven infusion of fentanyl: assessment of accuracy. Anesthesiology 1990; 73: 1082-90
28. Shafer SL, Varvel JR, Aziz N, Scott JC: Pharmacokinetics of fentanyl administered by computer-controlled infusion pump. Anesthesiology 1990; 73: 1091-102
29. Chaudhri S, White M, Kenny GN: Induction of anaesthesia with propofol using a target-controlled infusion system. Anaesthesia 1992; 47: 551-3
30. Glass PS, Glen JB, Kenny GN, Schuttler J, Shafer SL: Nomenclature for computer-assisted infusion devices. Anesthesiology 1997; 86: 1430-1

31. Glen JB: The development of 'Diprifusor': a TCI system for propofol. Anaesthesia 1998; 53 Suppl 1: 13-21
32. Gray JM, Kenny GN: Development of the technology for 'Diprifusor' TCI systems. Anaesthesia 1998; 53 Suppl 1: 22-27
33. Taylor I, White M, Kenny GN: Assessment of the value and pattern of use of a target controlled propofol infusion system. International Journal of Clinical Monitoring and Computing 1993; 10: 175-180
34. Russell D, Wilkes MP, Hunter SC, Glen JB, Hutton P, Kenny GN: Manual compared with target-controlled infusion of propofol. Br J Anaesth 1995; 75: 562-6
35. Glen JB: Quality of anaesthesia during spontaneous respiration: a proposed scoring system. Anaesthesia 1991; 46: 1081-1082
36. Struys M, Versichelen L, Rolly G: Influence of pre-anaesthetic medication on target propofol concentration using a 'Diprifusor' TCI system during ambulatory surgery. Anaesthesia 1998; 53 Suppl 1:68-71: 68-71
37. Barvais L, Rausin I, Glen JB, Hunter SC, D'Hulster D, Cantraine F, D'Hollander A: Administration of propofol by target-controlled infusion in patients undergoing coronary artery surgery. J.Cardiothorac.Vasc.Anesth. 1996; 10: 877-883
38. Swinhoe CF, Peacock JE, Reilly CS: Evaluation of the accuracy of the 'Diprifusor'. European Journal of Anaesthesiology – Supplement 1995; 10: 84
39. Richards AL, Orton JK, Gregory MJ: Influence of ventilatory mode on target concentrations required for anaesthesia using a 'Diprifusor' TCI system. Anaesthesia 1998; 53 Suppl 1: 77-81
40. Servin FS, Marchand-Maillet F, Desmonts JM: Influence of analgesic supplementation on the target propofol concentrations for anaesthesia with 'Diprifusor' TCI. Anaesthesia 1998; 53 Suppl 1: 72-76
41. Servin FS: TCI compared with manually controlled infusion of propofol: a multicentre study. Anaesthesia 1998; 53 Suppl 1:82-6: 82-86
42. Marsh B, White M, Morton N, Kenny GN: Pharmacokinetic model driven infusion of propofol in children. Br.J.Anaesth. 1991; 67: 41-48
43. Gepts E, Camu F, Cockshott ID, Douglas EJ: Disposition of propofol administered as constant rate intravenous infusions in humans. Anesthesia and Analgesia 1987; 66: 1256-1263
44. Schuttler J, Ihmsen H: Population pharmacokinetics of propofol: a multicenter study. Anesthesiology 2000; 92: 727-738
45. Schnider TW, Minto CF, Gambus PL, Andresen C, Goodale DB, Shafer SL, Youngs EJ: The influence of method of administration and covariates on the pharmacokinetics of propofol in adult volunteers. Anesthesiology 1998; 88: 1170-82

46. Saint-Maurice C, Cockshott ID, Douglas EJ, Richard MO, Harmey JL: Pharmacokinetics of propofol in young children after a single dose. Br J Anaesth 1989; 63: 667-670
47. Murat I, Billard V, Vernois J, Zaouter M, Marsol P, Souron R, Farinotti R: Pharmacokinetics of propofol after a single dose in children aged 1-3 years with minor burns. Comparison of three data analysis approaches. Anesthesiology 1996; 84: 526-32
48. Kataria BK, Ved SA, Nicodemus HF, Hoy GR, Lea D, Dubois MY, Mandema JW, Shafer SL: The pharmacokinetics of propofol in children using three different data analysis approaches. Anesthesiology 1994; 80: 104-22
49. Absalom A, Amutike D, Lal A, White M, Kenny GN: Accuracy of the 'Paedfusor' in children undergoing cardiac surgery or catheterization. Br J Anaesth 2003; 91: 507-13
50. Short TG, Aun CS, Tan P, Wong J, Tam YH, Oh TE: A prospective evaluation of pharmacokinetic model controlled infusion of propofol in paediatric patients. Br J Anaesth 1994; 72: 302-306
51. Dershwitz M, Hoke JF, Rosow CE, Michalowski P, Connors PM, Muir KT, Dienstag JL: Pharmacokinetics and pharmacodynamics of remifentanil in volunteer subjects with severe liver disease. Anesthesiology 1996; 84: 812-20
52. Hoke JF, Shlugman D, Dershwitz M, Michalowski P, Malthouse-Dufore S, Connors PM, Martel D, Rosow CE, Muir KT, Rubin N, Glass PS: Pharmacokinetics and pharmacodynamics of remifentanil in persons with renal failure compared with healthy volunteers. Anesthesiology 1997; 87: 533-541
53. Minto CF, Schnider TW, Egan TD, Youngs E, Lemmens HJ, Gambus PL, Billard V, Hoke JF, Moore KH, Hermann DJ, Muir KT, Mandema JW, Shafer SL: Influence of age and gender on the pharmacokinetics and pharmacodynamics of remifentanil. I. Model development. Anesthesiology 1997; 86: 10-23
54. Minto CF, Schnider TW, Shafer SL: Pharmacokinetics and pharmacodynamics of remifentanil. II. Model application. Anesthesiology 1997; 86: 24-33
55. Gepts E, Shafer SL, Camu F, Stanski DR, Woestenborghs R, Van Peer A, Heykants JJ: Linearity of pharmacokinetics and model estimation of sufentanil. Anesthesiology 1995; 83: 1194-204
56. Bovill JG, Sebel PS, Blackburn CL, Oei-Lim V, Heykants JJ: The pharmacokinetics of sufentanil in surgical patients. Anesthesiology 1984; 61: 502-506
57. Helmers JH, van Leeuwen L, Zuurmond WW: Sufentanil pharmacokinetics in young adult and elderly surgical patients. European Journal of Anaesthesiology 1994; 11: 181-185
58. Camu F, Gepts E, Rucquoi M, Heykants J: Pharmacokinetics of alfentanil in man. Anesth Analg 1982; 61: 657-61

59. Bower S, Hull CJ: Comparative pharmacokinetics of fentanyl and alfentanil. Br J Anaesth 1982; 54: 871-7
60. Chauvin M, Bonnet F, Montembault C, Levron JC, Viars P: The influence of hepatic plasma flow on alfentanil plasma concentration plateaus achieved with an infusion model in humans: measurement of alfentanil hepatic extraction coefficient. Anesthesia and Analgesia 1986; 65: 999-1003
61. Bovill JG, Sebel PS, Blackburn CL, Heykants J: The pharmacokinetics of alfentanil (R39209): a new opioid analgesic. Anesthesiology 1982; 57: 439-43
62. Helmers H, Van Peer A, Woestenborghs R, Noorduin H, Heykants J: Alfentanil kinetics in the elderly. Clin Pharmacol Ther 1984; 36: 239-43
63. Maitre PO, Vozeh S, Heykants J, Thomson DA, Stanski DR: Population pharmacokinetics of alfentanil: the average dose – plasma concentration relationship and interindividual variability in patients. Anesthesiology 1987; 66: 3-12
64. Roerig DL, Kotrly KJ, Vucins EJ, Ahlf SB, Dawson CA, Kampine JP: First pass uptake of fentanyl, meperidine, and morphine in the human lung. Anesthesiology 1987; 67: 466-72
65. Egan TD, Lemmens HJ, Fiset P, Hermann DJ, Muir KT, Stanski DR, Shafer SL: The pharmacokinetics of the new short-acting opioid remifentanil (GI87084B) in healthy adult male volunteers. Anesthesiology 1993; 79: 881-892
66. Hughes MA, Glass PS, Jacobs JR: Context-sensitive half-time in multicompartment pharmacokinetic models for intravenous anesthetic drugs. Anesthesiology 1992; 76: 334-341
67. McClain DA, Hug CC, Jr.: Intravenous fentanyl kinetics. Clin Pharmacol Ther 1980; 28: 106-14
68. Hudson RJ, Thomson IR, Cannon JE, Friesen RM, Meatherall RC: Pharmacokinetics of fentanyl in patients undergoing abdominal aortic surgery. Anesthesiology 1986; 64: 334-8
69. Scott JC, Stanski DR: Decreased fentanyl and alfentanil dose requirements with age. A simultaneous pharmacokinetic and pharmacodynamic evaluation. J.Pharmacol.Exp.Ther. 1987; 240: 159-166
70. Shibutani K, Inchiosa MA, Jr., Sawada K, Bairamian M: Accuracy of pharmacokinetic models for predicting plasma fentanyl concentrations in lean and obese surgical patients: derivation of dosing weight ("pharmacokinetic mass"). Anesthesiology 2004; 101: 603-13
71. Nagels W, Demeyere R, Van Hemelrijck J, Vandenbussche E, Gijbels K, Vandermeersch E: Evaluation of the neuroprotective effects of S(+)-ketamine during open-heart surgery. Anesthesia and Analgesia 2004; 98: 1595-603, table

72. Koppert W, Sittl R, Scheuber K, Alsheimer M, Schmelz M, Schuttler J: Differential modulation of remifentanil-induced analgesia and postinfusion hyperalgesia by S-ketamine and clonidine in humans. Anesthesiology 2003; 99: 152-9
73. Bell RF, Dahl JB, Moore RA, Kalso E: Perioperative ketamine for acute postoperative pain. Cochrane Database Syst Rev 2006: CD004603
74. Bourgoin A, Albanese J, Leone M, Sampol-Manos E, Viviand X, Martin C: Effects of sufentanil or ketamine administered in target-controlled infusion on the cerebral hemodynamics of severely brain-injured patients. Crit Care Med 2005; 33: 1109-13
75. Hijazi Y, Bodonian C, Bolon M, Salord F, Boulieu R: Pharmacokinetics and haemodynamics of ketamine in intensive care patients with brain or spinal cord injury. Br J Anaesth 2003; 90: 155-60
76. White M, de Graaff P, Renshof B, van Kan E, Dzoljic M: Pharmacokinetics of S(+) ketamine derived from target controlled infusion. Br J Anaesth 2006; 96: 330-4
77. Gray C, Swinhoe CF, Myint Y, Mason D: Target controlled infusion of ketamine as analgesia for TIVA with propofol. Can J Anaesth 1999; 46: 957-61
78. Katoh T, Suzuki A, Ikeda K: Electroencephalographic derivatives as a tool for predicting the depth of sedation and anesthesia induced by sevoflurane. Anesthesiology 1998; 88: 642-650
79. Luginbuhl M, Gerber A, Schnider TW, Petersen-Felix S, Arendt-Nielsen L, Curatolo M: Modulation of remifentanil-induced analgesia, hyperalgesia, and tolerance by small-dose ketamine in humans. Anesth Analg 2003; 96: 726-32
80. Rogers R, Wise RG, Painter DJ, Longe SE, Tracey I: An investigation to dissociate the analgesic and anesthetic properties of ketamine using functional magnetic resonance imaging. Anesthesiology 2004; 100: 292-301
81. Honey RA, Turner DC, Honey GD, Sharar SR, Kumaran D, Pomarol-Clotet E, McKenna P, Sahakian BJ, Robbins TW, Fletcher PC: Subdissociative dose ketamine produces a deficit in manipulation but not maintenance of the contents of working memory. Neuropsychopharmacology 2003; 28: 2037-44
82. Honey RA, Honey GD, O'Loughlin C, Sharar SR, Kumaran D, Bullmore ET, Menon DK, Donovan T, Lupson VC, Bisbrown-Chippendale R, Fletcher PC: Acute ketamine administration alters the brain responses to executive demands in a verbal working memory task: an FMRI study. Neuropsychopharmacology 2004; 29: 1203-14
83. Honey GD, O'Loughlin C, Turner DC, Pomarol-Clotet E, Corlett PR, Fletcher PC: The effects of a subpsychotic dose of ketamine on recognition and source memory for agency: implications for pharmacological modelling of core symptoms of schizophrenia. Neuropsychopharmacology 2006; 31: 413-23

84. Honey GD, Honey RA, Sharar SR, Turner DC, Pomarol-Clotet E, Kumaran D, Simons JS, Hu X, Rugg MD, Bullmore ET, Fletcher PC: Impairment of specific episodic memory processes by sub-psychotic doses of ketamine: the effects of levels of processing at encoding and of the subsequent retrieval task. Psychopharmacology (Berl) 2005; 181: 445-57
85. Honey GD, Honey RA, O'Loughlin C, Sharar SR, Kumaran D, Suckling J, Menon DK, Sleator C, Bullmore ET, Fletcher PC: Ketamine disrupts frontal and hippocampal contribution to encoding and retrieval of episodic memory: an fMRI study. Cereb Cortex 2005; 15: 749-59
86. Corlett PR, Honey GD, Aitken MR, Dickinson A, Shanks DR, Absalom AR, Lee M, Pomarol-Clotet E, Murray GK, McKenna PJ, Robbins TW, Bullmore ET, Fletcher PC: Frontal responses during learning predict vulnerability to the psychotogenic effects of ketamine: linking cognition, brain activity, and psychosis. Arch Gen Psychiatry 2006; 63: 611-21
87. Pomarol-Clotet E, Honey GD, Murray GK, Corlett PR, Absalom AR, Lee M, McKenna PJ, Bullmore ET, Fletcher PC: Psychological effects of ketamine in healthy volunteers. Phenomenological study. Br J Psychiatry 2006; 189: 173-9
88. Domino EF, Zsigmond EK, Domino LE, Domino KE, Kothary SP, Domino SE: Plasma levels of ketamine and two of its metabolites in surgical patients using a gas chromatographic mass fragmentographic assay. Anesth Analg 1982; 61: 87-92
89. Domino EF, Domino SE, Smith RE, Domino LE, Goulet JR, Domino KE, Zsigmond EK: Ketamine kinetics in unmedicated and diazepam-premedicated subjects. Clin Pharmacol Ther 1984; 36: 645-53
90. Geisslinger G, Hering W, Thomann P, Knoll R, Kamp HD, Brune K: Pharmacokinetics and pharmacodynamics of ketamine enantiomers in surgical patients using a stereoselective analytical method. Br J Anaesth 1993; 70: 666-671
91. Geisslinger G, Hering W, Kamp HD, Vollmers KO: Pharmacokinetics of ketamine enantiomers. Br J Anaesth 1995; 75: 506-507
92. Clements JA, Nimmo WS: Pharmacokinetics and analgesic effect of ketamine in man. Br J Anaesth 1981; 53: 27-30
93. Varvel JR, Donoho DL, Shafer SL: Measuring the predictive performance of computer-controlled infusion pumps. J Pharmacokinet Biopharm 1992; 20: 63-94
94. Schuttler J, Kloos S, Schwilden H, Stoeckel H: Total intravenous anaesthesia with propofol and alfentanil by computer-assisted infusion. Anaesthesia 1988; 43 Suppl: 2-7
95. Glass PJA, Jacobs JR, Reves JG, Miller RD: Intravenous drug delivery, Anesthesia. New York, Churchill Livingstone, 1990, pp 367
96. Frei FJ, Zbinden AM, Thomson DA, Rieder HU: Is the end-tidal partial pressure of isoflurane a good predictor of its arterial partial pressure? Br J Anaesth 1991; 66: 331-9

97. Dwyer RC, Fee JP, Howard PJ, Clarke RS: Arterial washin of halothane and isoflurane in young and elderly adult patients. Br J Anaesth 1991; 66: 572-9
98. Coetzee JF, Glen JB, Wium CA, Boshoff L: Pharmacokinetic model selection for target controlled infusions of propofol. Assessment of three parameter sets. Anesthesiology 1995; 82: 1328-45
99. Swinhoe CF, Peacock JE, Glen JB, Reilly CS: Evaluation of the predictive performance of a 'Diprifusor' TCI system. Anaesthesia 1998; 53 Suppl 1: 61-7
100. Barvais L, Rausin I, Glen JB, Hunter SC, D'Hulster D, Cantraine F, D'Hollander A: Administration of propofol by target-controlled infusion in patients undergoing coronary artery surgery. J Cardiothorac Vasc Anesth 1996; 10: 877-883
101. Davidson JA, Macleod AD, Howie JC, White M, Kenny GN: Effective concentration 50 for propofol with and without 67% nitrous oxide. Acta Anaesthesiologica Scandinavica 1993; 37: 458-464
102. Mertens MJ, Engbers FH, Burm AG, Vuyk J: Predictive performance of computer-controlled infusion of remifentanil during propofol/remifentanil anaesthesia. Br J Anaesth 2003; 90: 132-141
103. Barvais L, Heitz D, Schmartz D, Maes V, Coussaert E, Cantraine F, d'Hollander A: Pharmacokinetic model-driven infusion of sufentanil and midazolam during cardiac surgery: assessment of the prospective predictive accuracy and the quality of anesthesia. J Cardiothorac Vasc Anesth 2000; 14: 402-8
104. Pandin PC, Cantraine F, Ewalenko P, Deneu SC, Coussaert E, d'Hollander AA: Predictive accuracy of target-controlled propofol and sufentanil coinfusion in long-lasting surgery. Anesthesiology 2000; 93: 653-661
105. Hudson RJ, Henderson BT, Thomson IR, Moon M, Peterson MD: Pharmacokinetics of sufentanil in patients undergoing coronary artery bypass graft surgery. J.Cardiothorac.Vasc.Anesth. 2001; 15: 693-699
106. Slepchenko G, Simon N, Goubaux B, Levron JC, Le Moing JP, Raucoules-Aime M: Performance of target-controlled sufentanil infusion in obese patients. Anesthesiology 2003; 98: 65-73
107. Maitre PO, Ausems ME, Vozeh S, Stanski DR: Evaluating the accuracy of using population pharmacokinetic data to predict plasma concentrations of alfentanil. Anesthesiology 1988; 68: 59-67
108. Barvais L, d Hollander A, Schmartz D, Hendrice C, Cantraine F, Coussaert E: Predictive accuracy of alfentanil infusion in coronary artery surgery: a prebypass study in middle-aged and elderly patients. J.Cardiothorac.Vasc.Anesth. 1994; 8: 278-283
109. Absalom AR, Lee M, Menon DK, Sharar SR, De Smet T, Halliday J, Ogden M, Corlett P, Honey GD, Fletcher PC: Predictive performance of the Domino, Hijazi, and Clements models during low-dose target-controlled ketamine infusions in healthy volunteers. Br J Anaesth 2007; 98: 615-23

110. Matot I, Neely CF, Katz RY, Neufeld GR: Pulmonary uptake of propofol in cats. Effect of fentanyl and halothane. Anesthesiology 1993; 78: 1157-1165

111. Baker MT, Chadam MV, Ronnenberg WC, Jr.: Inhibitory effects of propofol on cytochrome P450 activities in rat hepatic microsomes. Anesthesia and Analgesia 1993; 76: 817-821

112. Mertens MJ, Vuyk J, Olofsen E, Bovill JG, Burm AG: Propofol alters the pharmacokinetics of alfentanil in healthy male volunteers. Anesthesiology 2001; 94: 949-957

113. Cockshott ID, Briggs LP, Douglas EJ, White M: Pharmacokinetics of propofol in female patients. Studies using single bolus injections. Br J Anaesth 1987; 59: 1103-1110

114. Pavlin DJ, Coda B, Shen DD, Tschanz J, Nguyen Q, Schaffer R, Donaldson G, Jacobson RC, Chapman CR: Effects of combining propofol and alfentanil on ventilation, analgesia, sedation, and emesis in human volunteers. Anesthesiology 1996; 84: 23-37

115. Bouillon T, Bruhn J, Radu-Radulescu L, Andresen C, Cohane C, Shafer SL: A model of the ventilatory depressant potency of remifentanil in the non-steady state. Anesthesiology 2003; 99: 779-787

116. Egan TD: Remifentanil pharmacokinetics and pharmacodynamics. A preliminary appraisal. Clinical Pharmacokinetics 1995; 29: 80-94

117. Leslie K, Crankshaw DP: Lean tissue mass is a useful predictor of induction dose requirements for propofol. Anaesth.Intensive Care 1991; 19: 57-60

118. Wulfsohn NL, Joshi CW: Thiopentone dosage based on lean body mass. Br J Anaesth 1969; 41: 516-521

119. Beemer GH, Bjorksten AR, Crankshaw DP: Pharmacokinetics of atracurium during continuous infusion. Br J Anaesth 1990; 65: 668-674

120. Egan TD, Huizinga B, Gupta SK, Jaarsma RL, Sperry RJ, Yee JB, Muir KT: Remifentanil pharmacokinetics in obese versus lean patients. Anesthesiology 1998; 89: 562-573

121. Abernethy DR, Greenblatt DJ, Divoll M, Harmatz JS, Shader RI: Alterations in drug distribution and clearance due to obesity. J.Pharmacol.Exp.Ther. 1981; 217: 681-685

122. James W: Research on obesity. London, Her Majesty's Stationary Office, 1976

123. Billard V, Gambus PL, Chamoun N, Stanski DR, Shafer SL: A comparison of spectral edge, delta power, and bispectral index as EEG measures of alfentanil, propofol, and midazolam drug effect. Clinical Pharmacology & Therapeutics 1997; 61: 45-58

124. Struys MM, De Smet T, Depoorter B, Versichelen LF, Mortier EP, Dumortier FJ, Shafer SL, Rolly G: Comparison of plasma compartment versus two methods for effect compartment – controlled target-controlled infusion for propofol. Anesthesiology 2000; 92: 399-406

125. Scott JC, Ponganis KV, Stanski DR: EEG quantitation of narcotic effect: the comparative pharmacodynamics of fentanyl and alfentanil. Anesthesiology 1985; 62: 234-241
126. Scott JC, Cooke JE, Stanski DR: Electroencephalographic quantitation of opioid effect: comparative pharmacodynamics of fentanyl and sufentanil. Anesthesiology 1991; 74: 34-42
127. Shafer SL, Varvel JR: Pharmacokinetics, pharmacodynamics, and rational opioid selection. Anesthesiology 1991; 74: 53-63
128. Irwin MG, Thompson N, Kenny GN: Patient-maintained propofol sedation. Assessment of a target-controlled infusion system. Anaesthesia 1997; 52: 525-530
129. Murdoch JA, Kenny GN: Patient-maintained propofol sedation as premedication in day-case surgery: assessment of a target-controlled system. Br J Anaesth 1999; 82: 429-431
130. Murdoch J, Grant S, Kenny G: Safety of patient-maintained propofol sedation using a target- controlled system in healthy volunteers. Br J Anaesth 2000; 85: 299-301
131. Henderson F, Absalom AR, Kenny GN: Patient-maintained propofol sedation: a follow up safety study using a modified system in volunteers. Anaesthesia 2002; 57: 387-90
132. McMurray TJ, Johnston JR, Milligan KR, Grant IS, Mackenzie SJ, Servin F, Janvier G, Glen JB: Propofol sedation using Diprifusor target-controlled infusion in adult intensive care unit patients. Anaesthesia 2004; 59: 636-641
133. Schuttler J, Stoeckel H, Schwilden H: Pharmacokinetic and pharmacodynamic modelling of propofol ('Diprivan') in volunteers and surgical patients. Postgrad Med J 1985; 61 Suppl 3: 53-4
134. Struys MM, Vereecke H, Moerman A, Jensen EW, Verhaeghen D, De Neve N, Dumortier FJ, Mortier EP: Ability of the bispectral index, autoregressive modelling with exogenous input-derived auditory evoked potentials, and predicted propofol concentrations to measure patient responsiveness during anesthesia with propofol and remifentanil. Anesthesiology 2003; 99: 802-812
135. Stuart PC, Stott SM, Millar A, Kenny GN, Russell D: Cp50 of propofol with and without nitrous oxide 67%. Br J Anaesth 2000; 84: 638-639
136. Leslie K, Sessler DI, Schroeder M, Walters K: Propofol blood concentration and the Bispectral Index predict suppression of learning during propofol/epidural anesthesia in volunteers. Anesthesia & Analgesia 1995; 81: 1269-1274
137. Mertens MJ, Olofsen E, Engbers FH, Burm AG, Bovill JG, Vuyk J: Propofol reduces perioperative remifentanil requirements in a synergistic manner: response surface modeling of perioperative remifentanil-propofol interactions. Anesthesiology 2003; 99: 347-359
138. Bailey JM, Schwieger IM, Hug CC, Jr.: Evaluation of sufentanil anesthesia obtained by a computer-controlled infusion for cardiac surgery. Anesthesia and Analgesia 1993; 76: 247-252

139. Glass P, Shafer S, Reves J: Intravenous drug delivery systems, Anesthesia, 5th Edition. Edited by Miller R. New York, Churchill-Livingstone, 2000, pp 377-411
140. Ausems ME, Hug CC: Plasma concentrations of alfentanil required to supplement nitrous oxide anaesthesia for lower abdominal surgery. Br J Anaesth 1983; 55 Suppl 2: 191S-197S
141. Ausems ME, Stanski DR, Hug CC: An evaluation of the accuracy of pharmacokinetic data for the computer assisted infusion of alfentanil. Br J Anaesth 1985; 57: 1217-25
142. Ausems ME, Hug CC, Jr., Stanski DR, Burm AG: Plasma concentrations of alfentanil required to supplement nitrous oxide anesthesia for general surgery. Anesthesiology 1986; 65: 362-73
143. Vuyk J, Lim T, Engbers FH, Burm AG, Vletter AA, Bovill JG: Pharmacodynamics of alfentanil as a supplement to propofol or nitrous oxide for lower abdominal surgery in female patients. Anesthesiology 1993; 78: 1036-1045
144. Katoh T, Kobayashi S, Suzuki A, Iwamoto T, Bito H, Ikeda K: The effect of fentanyl on sevoflurane requirements for somatic and sympathetic responses to surgical incision. Anesthesiology 1999; 90: 398-405
145. McEwan AI, Smith C, Dyar O, Goodman D, Smith LR, Glass PS: Isoflurane minimum alveolar concentration reduction by fentanyl. Anesthesiology 1993; 78: 864-869
146. Smith C, McEwan AI, Jhaveri R, Wilkinson M, Goodman D, Smith LR, Canada AT, Glass PS: The interaction of fentanyl on the Cp50 of propofol for loss of consciousness and skin incision. Anesthesiology 1994; 81: 820-828
147. Westmoreland CL, Sebel PS, Gropper A: Fentanyl or alfentanil decreases the minimum alveolar anesthetic concentration of isoflurane in surgical patients. Anesthesia and Analgesia 1994; 78: 23-28
148. Conway DH, Hasan SK, Simpson ME: Target-controlled propofol requirements at induction of anaesthesia: effect of remifentanil and midazolam. European Journal of Anaesthesiology 2002; 19: 580-584
149. Cressey DM, Claydon P, Bhaskaran NC, Reilly CS: Effect of midazolam pretreatment on induction dose requirements of propofol in combination with fentanyl in younger and older adults. Anaesthesia 2001; 56: 108-113
150. Jones NA, Elliott S, Knight J: A comparison between midazolam co-induction and propofol predosing for the induction of anaesthesia in the elderly. Anaesthesia 2002; 57: 649-653
151. Richards MJ, Skues MA, Jarvis AP, Prys-Roberts C: Total i.v. anaesthesia with propofol and alfentanil: dose requirements for propofol and the effect of premedication with clonidine. Br J Anaesth 1990; 65: 157-163
152. Johansen JW, Flaishon R, Sebel PS: Esmolol reduces anesthetic requirement for skin incision during propofol/nitrous oxide/morphine anesthesia. Anesthesiology 1997; 86: 364-371

153. Korpinen R, Saarnivaara L, Siren K, Sarna S: Modification of the haemodynamic responses to induction of anaesthesia and tracheal intubation with alfentanil, esmolol and their combination. Canadian Journal of Anaesthesia 1995; 42: 298-304
154. Smith I, Van Hemelrijck J, White PF: Efficacy of esmolol versus alfentanil as a supplement to propofol-nitrous oxide anesthesia. Anesthesia and Analgesia 1991; 73: 540-546
155. Wilson ES, McKinlay S, Crawford JM, Robb HM: The influence of esmolol on the dose of propofol required for induction of anaesthesia. Anaesthesia 2004; 59: 122-126
156. Vuyk J, Engbers FH, Burm AL, Vletter AA, Griever GE, Olofsen E, Bovill JG: Pharmacodynamic interaction between propofol and alfentanil when given for induction of anesthesia. Anesthesiology 1996; 84: 288-299
157. Vuyk J, Mertens MJ, Olofsen E, Burm AG, Bovill JG: Propofol anesthesia and rational opioid selection: determination of optimal EC50-EC95 propofol-opioid concentrations that assure adequate anesthesia and a rapid return of consciousness. Anesthesiology 1997; 87: 1549-62
158. Nieuwenhuijs DJ, Olofsen E, Romberg RR, Sarton E, Ward D, Engbers F, Vuyk J, Mooren R, Teppema LJ, Dahan A: Response surface modeling of remifentanil-propofol interaction on cardiorespiratory control and bispectral index. Anesthesiology 2003; 98: 312-322
159. Bouillon TW, Bruhn J, Radulescu L, Andresen C, Shafer TJ, Cohane C, Shafer SL: Pharmacodynamic interaction between propofol and remifentanil regarding hypnosis, tolerance of laryngoscopy, bispectral index, and electroencephalographic approximate entropy. Anesthesiology 2004; 100: 1353-1372
160. Roberts FL, Dixon J, Lewis GT, Tackley RM, Prys-Roberts C: Induction and maintenance of propofol anaesthesia. A manual infusion scheme. Anaesthesia 1988; 43 Suppl: 14-17
161. Munoz HR, Guerrero ME, Brandes V, Cortinez LI: Effect of timing of morphine administration during remifentanil-based anaesthesia on early recovery from anaesthesia and postoperative pain. Br J Anaesth 2002; 88: 814-818
162. Thurlow JA, Laxton CH, Dick A, Waterhouse P, Sherman L, Goodman NW: Remifentanil by patient-controlled analgesia compared with intramuscular meperidine for pain relief in labour. Br J Anaesth 2002; 88: 374-378
163. McCarroll CP, Paxton LD, Elliott P, Wilson DB: Use of remifentanil in a patient with peripartum cardiomyopathy requiring Caesarean section. Br J Anaesth 2001; 86: 135-138
164. Blair JM, Hill DA, Fee JP: Patient-controlled analgesia for labour using remifentanil: a feasibility study. Br J Anaesth 2001; 87: 415-420
165. Gallagher G, Rae CP, Kenny GN, Kinsella J: The use of a target-controlled infusion of alfentanil to provide analgesia for burn dressing changes A dose finding study. Anaesthesia 2000; 55: 1159-1163

166. Irwin MG, Jones RD, Visram AR, Kenny GN: Patient-controlled alfentanil. Target-controlled infusion for postoperative analgesia. Anaesthesia 1996; 51: 427-430
167. Turfrey DJ, Ray DA, Sutcliffe NP, Ramayya P, Kenny GN, Scott NB: Thoracic epidural anaesthesia for coronary artery bypass graft surgery. Effects on postoperative complications. Anaesthesia 1997; 52: 1090-1095
168. Checketts MR, Gilhooly CJ, Kenny GN: Patient-maintained analgesia with target controlled alfentanil after cardiac surgery: a comparison with morphine PCA. Br J Anaesth 1998; 80: 748-751
169. Schraag S, Kenny GN, Mohl U, Georgieff M: Patient-maintained remifentanil target-controlled infusion for the transition to early postoperative analgesia. Br J Anaesth 1998; 81: 365-368
170. Manninen PH, Balki M, Lukitto K, Bernstein M: Patient satisfaction with awake craniotomy for tumor surgery: a comparison of remifentanil and fentanyl in conjunction with propofol. Anesth Analg 2006; 102: 237-42
171. Lang E, Kapila A, Shlugman D, Hoke JF, Sebel PS, Glass PS: Reduction of isoflurane minimal alveolar concentration by remifentanil. Anesthesiology 1996; 85: 721-728
172. Albertin A, Casati A, Bergonzi P, Fano G, Torri G: Effects of two target-controlled concentrations (1 and 3 ng/ml) of remifentanil on MAC(BAR) of sevoflurane. Anesthesiology 2004; 100: 255-9
173. Albertin A, Casati A, Bergonzi PC, Moizo E, Lombardo F, Torri G: The effect of adding nitrous oxide on MAC of sevoflurane combined with two target-controlled concentrations of remifentanil in women. Eur J Anaesthesiol 2005; 22: 431-7
174. Billard V, Servin F, Guignard B, Junke E, Bouverne MN, Hedouin M, Chauvin M: Desflurane-remifentanil-nitrous oxide anaesthesia for abdominal surgery: optimal concentrations and recovery features. Acta Anaesthesiol Scand 2004; 48: 355-64
175. Albertin A, Dedola E, Bergonzi PC, Lombardo F, Fusco T, Torri G: The effect of adding two target-controlled concentrations (1-3 ng mL^{-1}) of remifentanil on MAC BAR of desflurane. Eur J Anaesthesiol 2006; 23: 510-6
176. Mortier E, Struys M, De Smet T, Versichelen L, Rolly G: Closed-loop controlled administration of propofol using bispectral analysis. Anaesthesia 1998; 53: 749-754
177. Leslie K, Absalom A, Kenny GN: Closed loop control of sedation for colonoscopy using the Bispectral Index. Anaesthesia 2002; 57: 693-7
178. Kenny GN, Mantzaridis H: Closed-loop control of propofol anaesthesia. Br.J.Anaesth. 1999; 83: 223-228
179. Struys MM, De Smet T, Versichelen LF, Van DV, Van den BR, Mortier EP: Comparison of closed-loop controlled administration of propofol using Bispectral Index as the controlled variable versus "standard practice" controlled administration. Anesthesiology 2001; 95: 6-17

180. Absalom AR, Sutcliffe N, Kenny GN: Closed-loop control of anesthesia using Bispectral index: performance assessment in patients undergoing major orthopedic surgery under combined general and regional anesthesia. Anesthesiology 2002; 96: 67-73

181. Absalom AR, Kenny GN: Closed-loop control of propofol anaesthesia using bispectral index: performance assessment in patients receiving computer-controlled propofol and manually controlled remifentanil infusions for minor surgery. Br J Anaesth 2003; 90: 737-41